State, Society, and Covid-19 in East Asia

This book elucidates state-society relations in East Asia during the COVID-19 pandemic from a comparative perspective.

Based on the findings of cross-national surveys in Japan, South Korea, and China, the book scrutinizes the dynamics of the state–society relationships in each country, examining trends of change in this relationship during the COVID-19 pandemic. Citizens' attitudes toward individual freedom, the state's anti-pandemic policies, vaccine hesitancy, and income redistribution policies across the three countries are compared revealing how public opinion in Japan, South Korea, and China during the COVID-19 pandemic provides a basis for understanding the complex relationship between state and society in East Asia.

Transcending national boundaries and uncovering citizens' evaluations of their domestic and neighboring countries' pandemic responses in East Asia, this book will be an indispensable resource for anyone interested in East Asian society and politics.

Taisuke Fujita is Associate Professor at Nagasaki University, Japan.

Hidehiro Yamamoto is Professor in the Institute of Humanities and Social Sciences at the University of Tsukuba, Japan.

Youngho Cho is Professor in Political Science at Sogang University in Seoul, South Korea.

Sang-Jin Han is Professor Emeritus at Seoul National University, South Korea.

Yida Zhai is Associate Professor of Political Science at the University of Tsukuba, Japan.

Routledge Contemporary Asian Societies

Routledge Contemporary Asian Societies provides an original and distinctive contribution to current debates on evolutions shaping societies, cultures, politics and media across North and South East Asia. It is interdisciplinary in its approach and the editors welcome proposals across the social sciences and humanities; from political, social, cultural and economic studies to gender, media, literature, anthropology, philosophy and religion.

Series Editors: Vanessa Frangville and Frederik Ponjaert, Research Centre on East Asia (EASt), Université libre de Bruxelles, Brussels, Belgium

China's Youth Culture and Collective Spaces
Creativity, Sociality, Identity and Resistance
Edited by Vanessa Frangville and Gwennaël Gaffric

History, Memory and Territorial Cults in the Highlands of Laos
The Past Inside the Present
Pierre Petit

China-Latin America and the Caribbean
Assessment and Outlook
Thierry Kellner and Sophie Wintgens

China's Green Consensus
Participation, Co-optation and Legitimation
Virginie Arantes

National Identity and Millennials in Northeast Asia
Power and Contestations in the Digital Age
Edited by Vanessa Frangville, Thierry Kellner and Frederik Ponjaert

State, Society, and Covid-19 in East Asia

Taisuke Fujita, Hidehiro Yamamoto, Youngho Cho, Sang-Jin Han and Yida Zhai

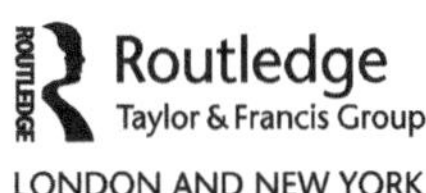
Routledge
Taylor & Francis Group
LONDON AND NEW YORK

First published 2025
by Routledge
4 Park Square, Milton Park, Abingdon, Oxon OX14 4RN

and by Routledge
605 Third Avenue, New York, NY 10158

Routledge is an imprint of the Taylor & Francis Group, an informa business

British Library Cataloguing-in-Publication Data
A catalogue record for this book is available from the British Library

ISBN: 978-1-032-79208-8 (hbk)
ISBN: 978-1-032-80062-2 (pbk)
ISBN: 978-1-003-49523-9 (ebk)

DOI: 10.4324/9781003495239

Typeset in Times New Roman
by Newgen Publishing UK

Contents

Figures

Tables

Contributors

Youngho Cho is Professor of Political Science at Sogang University in Seoul, South Korea. His research interests include Korean politics, democracy, and political culture. His works appear in *Asian Survey*, *Democratization*, and other journals.

Taisuke Fujita is Associate Professor at Nagasaki University, Japan. His research interests include international relations, comparative politics, public opinion, and comparative research methods. His work has been published in journals such as *Foreign Policy Analysis*, *Journal of East Asian Studies*, *Behaviormetrika*, and *Sociological Theory and Methods*.

Sang-Jin Han is Professor Emeritus at Seoul National University, South Korea. He lectured at Columbia University in New York and Peking University in Beijing. He is the author of *Asian Tradition and Cosmopolitan Politics* (2018), *Confucianism and Reflexive Modernity* (2020), and *Dialogue with Habermas* (2023 in Korean).

Gi-Woo Roh is a PhD candidate in Political Science at Sogang University in Seoul, South Korea. His research focuses on political behavior, public opinion, and youth politics.

Hidehiro Yamamoto is Professor in the Institute of Humanities and Social Sciences at the University of Tsukuba, Japan. He received his PhD in Literature at Tohoku University in 2003. His research focuses on political sociology, especially, state-society relationship, civil society, interest group, and political inequality. He is a coauthor of *Neighborhood Associations and Local Governance in Japan* (2014).

Yida Zhai is Associate Professor of Political Science at the University of Tsukuba, Japan. He studies political psychology, political sociology, and East Asian comparative politics/sociology. His research has appeared in *Contemporary Politics*, *Current Sociology*, *International Political Science Review*, and other Chinese journals.

1 Introduction

Yida Zhai

The COVID-19 Pandemic in China, Japan, and South Korea

Over five years have passed since the initial outbreak of COVID-19 in December 2019, and the pandemic has caused significant economic losses and a surge in the number of deaths worldwide. Undoubtedly, this is a global public health crisis, and no country is exempt from its disastrous influence. In response to the COVID-19 pandemic, each country adopted various countermeasures to control and prevent the spread of the virus, and great cross-national differences are observable in their anti-COVID-19 policies. Additionally, each country's citizenry has had a different response to the respective governments' policies. For example, American and European residents took to the streets to protest against local COVID-19 countermeasures, while in East Asian countries, there were only a few such protests, and people showed high levels of compliance with government anti-COVID-19 policies. This book focuses on three East Asian countries: Japan, the People's Republic of China (China), and the Republic of Korea (South Korea). People in these three countries hardly resisted the order to wear masks when outside of their home. They also followed the authorities' recommendations such as frequent hand washing, reducing social gatherings and activities, and social distancing. Further, they demonstrated a willingness to cooperate with local authorities in terms of tracking, testing, and isolating infected people or those who had close contact with confirmed cases. Moreover, they were less vigilant about the government's surveillance of their personal information during control of the viral spread (Kim, S. et al., 2020).

This chapter first reviews the COVID-19 pandemic situation and the government's response in the three focal countries. The outbreak was initially identified in mid-December 2019, and the earliest patients were linked to a seafood market in Wuhan, China (Wang et al., 2020; Zhao and Chen, 2020). According to the World Health Organization (WHO), on December 31, 2019, China reported a cluster of pneumonia cases detected in Wuhan, Hubei province. When some physicians attempted to raise the alarm regarding this infectious disease, they were prosecuted for spreading rumors. One of them, Li Wenliang, was reprimanded by the police (CGTN, 2020). Such actions were premised on the insistence of the head of the Wuhan Health Commission that evidence of human-to-human transmission

DOI: 10.4324/9781003495239-1

had not been found and that the risk of continued transmission was low (Ma, 2020; Zhang, 2020). On January 20, 2020, the prestigious physician Zhong Nanshan publicly claimed the existence of human-to-human transmission of the virus. The Chinese Lunar New Year fell on January 25 that year, and while the festive occasion typically witnesses great human mobility across China as people attend celebratory gatherings with family and friends, the central government intervened by implementing stringent measures to curb the spread of the virus. On January 23, 2020, Wuhan imposed lockdown, and no one was allowed to leave the area. However, this countermeasure was somewhat late in terms of effectiveness, as COVID-19 had already spread to all of China's provinces (Du et al., 2020; Zhao and Chen, 2020).

China implemented the zero-COVID policy. The leadership has propagandized China's superior performance with respect to the containment of the outbreak as evidence of the superiority of its political system compared to its democratic counterpart. The constituents of China's zero-COVID policy include large-scale nucleic acid testing, prompt contact tracing, and mandatory isolation and quarantine. Within China, "zero infection" has been set as a goal and a standard for the evaluation of local government's performance. The upward accountability that characterizes the Chinese political system motivates local officials to commit to the excessive imposition of lockdowns in pursuit of achieving zero-COVID. For instance, Wuhan, Xi'an, Changchun, Shenzhen, Shanghai, Chengdu, Lanzhou, and many other cities have had lockdowns. City authorities closed schools, factories, and public transport, canceled public events, stopped the movement of people in and out of the city, and issued blanket stay-home orders. Despite the Wuhan authorities' slow initial response, these aggressive measures have curbed the exponential increase in infections, and the number of cases in China has been relatively low compared to in other countries (WHO, 2022). While China sustained its stringent zero-COVID approach through the operationalization of its authoritarian political system, other countries that adopted a similar policy at some point have since transitioned to a state of coexistence with the virus, as unlike China, few countries are able to implement a long-term zero-tolerance COVID-19 policy (Anderson et al., 2020). However, with the emergence of the Omicron variant, the zero-COVID policy faced rising public discontent and a decline in political trust (Zeng, 2024; Zhai and Han, 2024). The political cost of lockdowns and enforced quarantine and a nationwide wave of protests terminated the zero-COVID policy in December 2022 (Guan et al., 2024; Zhai, 2023).

Japan is the host country of the 2020 Summer Olympics and Paralympic Games, and its anti-COVID-19 measures are balanced with the possible effects of such countermeasures on Olympics-related and economic activities. Japan reported its first COVID-19 case in mid-January 2020 and its second and third cases on January 24 and 25, 2020, respectively. The tourism industry was identified as the locus and agent of the viral spread, and bus/taxi drivers and tour guides were infected initially. The Diamond Princess incident was a critical early-stage issue that drew the world's attention. From January 28, 2020, to February 17, 2020, Japan evacuated more than 800 Japanese citizens from Wuhan on chartered flights (Shaw et al., 2020). On February 17, the Japanese government released consultation criteria for COVID-19 testing to guide the Japanese citizenry's pandemic response. On February 25, 2020, the government issued a fundamental action titled *Basic Policies for Novel Coronavirus Disease Control*, and on the same day, a cluster-response unit was established within the Ministry of Health, Labor, and Welfare (Shimizu and Negita, 2020).

Japan began implementing strict border control regulations in early February 2020 (Lu, 2020). Inbound visitors from China's Hubei province were required to complete 14 days of quarantine. Subsequently, over time, Japan also applied this policy to other high-risk countries. Given the risk of the spread of COVID-19, the Japanese government abruptly requested voluntary school closure in the last week of February 2020; the request found schools, teachers, and parents unprepared (Shaw et al., 2020). In the early stage, the Japanese authorities were criticized for their poor pandemic response, specifically a lack of transparency in terms of information disclosure and a low-efficiency case reporting and testing system (Chen, H. et al., 2021). The authorities encouraged people to wear masks, comply with social distancing, and work at home on a voluntary basis. However, the Japanese government did not implement any compulsory containment measures until April 2020. On April 7, 2020, then Japanese prime minister Shinzo Abe declared a pandemic-related state of emergency for Tokyo and six other prefectures (Saitama, Chiba, Kanagawa, Osaka, Hyogo, and Fukuoka). On April 16, 2020, the state of emergency was expanded beyond the seven abovementioned prefectures to encompass the entire nation with the intention of preventing the overwhelming of the medical system. The state of emergency helped significantly limit people's movement. Generally, Japan's response was a request for citizens' "self-restraint" and did not involve coercive measures (Ikeda, 2022: 2; Wright, 2021).

South Korea has a well-established legal system with respect to infectious disease control and prevention and has established a pan-governmental crisis management system that is supplemented and advanced based on experience with controlling past epidemics (Kim et al., 2021). On January 20, 2020, the Korea Disease Control and Prevention Agency (KDCA), formerly the Korea Centers for Disease Control and Prevention (KCDC), confirmed the first imported COVID-19 case (Shaw et al., 2020). In the face of the COVID-19 pandemic, South Korea did not impose city-wide lockdowns but rather adopted a "track, isolate, and treat" approach. The country quickly developed COVID-19 diagnostic kits and implemented large-scale testing to identify and isolate the infected population. Additionally, the KDCA directed treatment of infected people based on symptom severity. Patients with mild symptoms received treatment at home, while severe cases received intensive care while hospitalized. The KDCA also used personal information regarding travel history and economic transactions as well as CCTV footage to track close contacts of infected people (Kim, S. et al., 2020). Its strategy of rapid and extensive testing coupled with contact tracing proved effective in the early stage. Moreover, the government provided free smartphone apps to disseminate alerts and other pertinent information such as regarding online medical services for COVID-19 screening (Lu et al., 2020). South Korea has been recognized for its transparent information dissemination and efficient communication with the public in the context of public health crisis management (Chen, S. et al., 2021).

The Perspective of Changing State-Society Relations

This book explores state-society relations in China, Japan, and South Korea during the COVID-19 pandemic. The COVID-19 pandemic has, once again, brought the state into the spotlight (Woods et al., 2020). Although the pandemic has global influence, pandemic responses are local and contingent on different socioeconomic, political, and cultural contexts (Shaw et al., 2020). National anti-COVID-19 measures influence the pandemic's trajectory (Anderson et al., 2020). To handle this public health crisis, individual states are responsible for implementing measures such as setting restrictions, offering treatment and vaccination, and temporarily closing borders. At the micro-level, the crisis creates uncertainty and fear among populations. Individuals seek to reduce uncertainty and anxiety by increasing attachment to the state; hence, under crisis circumstances, they tolerate state intervention more than they would in normal times (Zhai, 2022). Meanwhile, the government provides people with some degree of security and safety in return for their loyalty and commitment (Druckman, 1994). As shown, state-society relations undergo change amid crises.

Crises create an opportunity for governments to expand their power. The COVID-19 pandemic is no exception. In many cases, the state has extended its power under the pretext of responding to the pandemic (Tsuji, 2022). For example, in many countries, the government tightened restrictions on daily activities, restricting people's freedoms and liberties (Anderson et al., 2020; Jia et al., 2021; Kupferschmidt and Cohen, 2020). Additionally, the state has used technology to track people's movement and contact with others, triggering controversy regarding privacy. Some infected people's personal information was leaked, causing privacy infringement and cyberbullying (Jung et al., 2020; Park et al., 2020). In China, Japan, and South Korea, emphasis is on the importance of political leadership and the government's policy decisions, as these constitute a determinant of the reactionary effects associated with the drawbacks of the anti-COVID-19 policy (Moon et al., 2021; Wang, 2020). Hence, this section will first review the role of the state in each of the three countries mentioned above.

The governments of China, Japan, and South Korea played a leading role in combating the COVID-19 pandemic. Each designed an overall anti-pandemic strategy, allocated resources, and guided private organizations to produce goods to meet medical and crisis mitigation needs (Wu et al., 2021). Specifically, China's pandemic response has featured a government-centered and top-down approach. China's authoritarian political system enabled the Chinese government to exercise magnificent power and mobilize resources to intervene in the pandemic. To contain the viral spread, the Chinese government first decided to lockdown Wuhan on January 23, 2020, and in the ten days that followed, all cities in Hubei province were locked down. Chinese leaders evidently favored the lockdown approach, and it was subsequently applied nationwide. On January 20, 2020, China established the State Council Joint Prevention and Control Mechanism, which was a leading and coordinating organization comprising 32 ministries and commissions. The State Council Joint Prevention and Control Mechanism was not only responsible for disease outbreak control and prevention but also coordinated production, transportation, and the supply of medical resources and living necessities. Additionally, the central government sent several "directing teams" headed by a vice premier or state councilor to the severely stricken cities to intensify local governmental supervision. Local officials with poor performance in anti-pandemic campaigns were removed from their posts and punished (Wang, 2020).

Regarding Japan's COVID-19 pandemic control, on January 30, 2020, the Japanese Cabinet decided to establish COVID-19 control headquarters as a cross-ministerial framework, headed by the prime minister, with the chief Cabinet secretary and the minister of health, labor, and welfare as co-deputy heads, and other ministers as members. An expert COVID-19 control committee was established on February 14, 2020, and 12 experts were appointed as members. According to some researchers, the role of experts in crisis management in Japan has been limited, since they neither made decisions nor were in charge of policy implementation (Moon et al., 2021). However, Shiroyama (2020) stressed that the expert COVID-19 control committee was not passive, as it released "situation analysis and recommendations" to the government and relevant stakeholders in society, which exerted an important influence in framing the Japanese government's agenda and the public's risk perception. After the revised Law on Special Measures Against New Influenza and Other Infectious Diseases came into effect on March 14, 2020, the COVID-19 control headquarters declared a state of emergency on April 7, 2020. Although Japan's policy was one of soft requests, under the state of emergency, a wide range of industries instituted temporary closures or reduced their operation time (Shiroyama, 2020). Admittedly, Japan's limited administrative and testing capacity has impeded the timely identification and isolation of infected persons (Inoue, 2020; Shimizu et al., 2020).

During the pandemic, the role of the state in South Korea has been as an efficient, experienced, and professional bureaucratic agency. The KDCA is an autonomous deputy ministerial-level agency specialized in epidemiological management (Moon, 2020). After the report of the first COVID-19-related death, the South Korean government assembled the Central Disaster Safety Control Tower under the prime minister's leadership. In fact, prior to the onset of the COVID-19 pandemic, the competitive bureaucracy was prepared to handle infectious diseases, as past experiences, such as responding to severe acute respiratory syndrome (SARS) in 2003 and Middle East Respiratory Syndrome (MERS) in 2015 and 2018, have been institutionalized (Im, 2020; Lee, S. et al., 2020). On February 4, 2020, the government promptly introduced a special entry procedure applicable to travelers from China, and on March 19, applicability of this procedure was expanded to travelers from all countries. As of April 1, 2020, all incoming travelers were required to undertake a 14-day self-quarantine (Jee, 2020). Further, as part of their quick response, the government scaled up the alert level to increase the public's attention to related matters. Within its 4-level national crisis management system, the government raised the alert level to 2 on January 20, to 3 on January 27, and to 4 on February 23, 2020. Moreover, the KDCA reintroduced enhanced entry screening for travelers from abroad and issued guidance to the public and local governments. Regarding treatment, as previously mentioned, the KDCA directed infected persons to different facilities depending on symptom severity. Patients with mild symptoms received treatment at community centers, and those with severe symptoms were hospitalized. This system ensured that confirmed cases received proper treatment and prevented the overwhelming of hospitals (Jee, 2020).

The other aspect of state-society relations is civil society. Civil society refers to the field comprising individuals and organizations that are not affiliated with the state and are not profit-seeking (Salamon and Sokolowski, 2004). The development of civil society differs significantly in the three focal countries. In China, the government is vigilant regarding civil society and worries that free development will threaten its authoritarian rule. Accordingly, it seeks to control civil society and bring all social organizations under its management (Kang and Heng, 2008). One mechanism for achieving this is the requirement that social organizations must satisfy a complicated registration procedure to obtain legal status in China. The purpose of such screening is to ensure that these organizations do not challenge the government. Hence, many autonomous grassroots social organizations have failed to clear screening and were thus deprived of legal status (Hsu and Hasmath, 2014). In China, civil society is not a sector that is independent of the state; rather, civil society must depend on and cooperate with the state to survive.

Civil society is an important force in Japanese society. Japanese civil society has a long history of providing social services. Although Japan's democratic political system enables a civil society that is independent of the state, compared with the confrontational state–society relations that exist in Western countries, Japanese civil society cooperates with rather than challenges the state, as evidenced by the relatively low incidence of confrontational social movements (Chiavacci and Obinger, 2018). In Japan, non-profit organizations (NPOs) were institutionalized under the 1998 NPO law (Ogawa, 2019). Under the new public governance framework, the Japanese state has established a collaborative relationship with civil society organizations regarding policy, incorporated into a structure that supports state goals (Ogawa, 2004, 2021). Some researchers have contended that Japanese civil society has had little opportunity to influence national policy (Pekkanen, 2006). However, a new and unprecedented wave of social and political protest movements resurged in the wake of the 2011 Fukushima nuclear accident (Machimura and Satoh, 2016). Among Japanese civil society's anti-nuclear movements, protesters demonstrated in front of the prime minister's residence every Friday. Additionally, in 2014 and 2015, Japanese civil society organized large-scale protests to oppose the Abe administration's new security bill legislation. Regarding Japanese youth activism, an organization called Students Emergency Action for Liberal Democracy (SEALDs) has been the most salient (Falch and Hammond, 2020; Kingston, 2015). Generally, the new wave of civic activism and street politics indicates that Japanese civil society has changed (Chiavacci and Obinger, 2018; Hasegawa, 2018; Oguma, 2016).

Civil society was a driving force in South Korea's democratization in the 1970s and 1980s. In the post-Korean War era, the authoritarian regime disallowed a strong civil society by oppressing its development. However, South Korean civil society was vibrant and resilient; three constituent groups—namely students, laborers, and the church—played a critical role in facilitating authoritarian breakdown and democratic transition in 1987 (Kim, S. 2000). This bottom-up transition model represents an alternative to the elitist paradigm (Fiori and Kim, 2018). After the democratic transition, the demise of the repressive state paved the way for citizens' engagement in the public sphere and for the mushrooming of nongovernmental organizations (NGOs) in South Korea (Kim, M. 2000). Participatory culture underlines South Korean democracy, suggesting substantial tension within state-society relations (Cho et al., 2019; Oh, 2012). Civil society contributes to identifying social problems that the state has undervalued and to sponsoring various reform efforts, such as campaigns for economic justice, gender equality, and environmental protection (Fiori and Kim, 2018). South Korea's strong civil society serves as a check on state abuse of power. In the post-transitional period, the politicization and ideological polarization of civil society have been a prominent characteristic of South Korea (Kim and Jeong, 2017).

In the three focal countries, civil society has assisted the government in combating the COVID-19 pandemic. NGOs have raised funds, amassed medical resources, disseminated pertinent information, and provided imperative social services, thereby enhancing social resilience to cope with the pandemic (Cai et al., 2021). However, differences exist across the three countries in terms of the interaction between the state and civil society amid the pandemic. Chinese civil society primarily played the role of mobilizing donated funds and medical resources. Given China's restrictive policies, all activities were state-supervised. Although grassroots NGOs are marginalized, they have outperformed the government in terms of managing donations and disseminating information. In Japan, collaboration between the government and civil society has been limited to neighborhood and residents' associations (Cai et al., 2021). In most cases, Japanese civil society acted independently, without collaborating with the government, specifically by fulfilling unmet demand for social services, holding conferences to report on shortcomings in the government's anti-COVID-19 policies, and offering policy recommendations (Cai et al., 2021). Compared to active governmental intervention in other countries, such as large-scale testing and contact tracing, Japan's public health COVID-19 response has depended heavily on its citizens' self-restraint (Ikeda, 2022: 2; Wright, 2021).

In South Korea's case, civil society significantly reinforced collaborative partnerships with governments, including information sharing, service provision, and administrative support. Public-private partnerships have functioned effectively in South Korea, enabling rapid approval of test kits, contact tracing, and the sensible allocation of medical resources (Choi, 2020; Kim et al., 2021). In combating COVID-19, South Korea has worked to secure civic engagement and voluntary participation within its citizenry and among social organizations (Lee, D. et al., 2020). The South Korean government even invited NGOs to emergency meetings.

Ultimately, the pandemic has enhanced the collaborative relationship between the state and civil society in South Korea (Cai et al., 2021).

Cross-National Comparative Studies and Datasets

Compared to Western nations, the total number of deaths per million inhabitants has remained low in China, Japan, and South Korea (WHO, 2022). Regarding their national COVID-19 response strategies, these three East Asian countries share many similarities but also differ in some ways. With respect to their core strategies, China and South Korea adopted containment, while Japan opted for a much softer option in mitigation (Chen, H. et al., 2021). For instance, the Japanese government's declaration of a state of emergency was essentially a symbolic gesture and was not concomitant with compulsory measures (Yan et al., 2020). In the case of South Korea, it is certainly true that, compared to China's aggressive and forceful measures, such as lockdowns, South Korea's strategy can be accurately described as an agile-adaptive approach (Moon, 2020).

Institutional arrangements and national cultural orientations are regarded as the two critical contextual factors that have influenced the observable cross-national variations in countries' control and prevention strategies (Yan et al., 2020). The combination of the culture and the government's countermeasures may account for the low fatality rates in China, Japan, and South Korea. This book focuses on these three countries for the following reasons. First, China, Japan, and South Korea share a Confucian cultural tradition that emphasizes respect for authorities and order, hierarchical relationships, and the maintenance of harmony and prioritizes the group before the self (Shin, 2012; Tu, 1996). Hence, in these three countries, individuals are not autonomous and independent in society, the "self" is a group-based conception, and interdependence with other members in groups is highly valued (Zhai, 2024). Cultural psychologists use the term "collectivist culture" to refer to the common cultural characteristics of China, Japan, and South Korea. Collectivist culture is distinct from the West's individualist culture, in which personal autonomy, independence, and achievements are encouraged (Kim et al., 1994; Kyriacou, 2016). Hence, collectivist cultural orientations may have promoted citizens' compliance with the government's anti-COVID-19 policies in these three countries.

Second, all three countries are developmental states (Cai et al., 2021), which means that the state plays a role in national development, specifically by intervening in industry investment and dominating economic planning (Woo-Cumings, 1999). The term "developmental state" has been used to explain the rapid growth of economic entities in East Asia. Strong states and social coalitions have been observed in these countries (Haggard, 2018). Government agencies in China, Japan, and South Korea have actively engaged in promoting national prosperity and public welfare. They have formulated industrial policies and fostered technological modernization. This developmental strategy in East Asia differs from the capitalist development model in Western countries, where private enterprises rather than governments are the primary drivers of economic development and technological advancement (Shin, 2012). Support for government intervention may distinguish these three East Asian countries from others in terms of COVID-19 control and prevention measures. The characteristics of a developmental state reveal a similarity in the three focal countries' state-society relations.

Third, there are differences among the three countries in terms of their political systems. Japan and South Korea are liberal democracies, while China is an authoritarian country. In democracies, the rule of law and checks and balances on power restrain the government's potential abuse of power. Hence, in democracies, with regard to the COVID-19 pandemic, efforts to curtail the outbreak must be balanced with respect for citizens' democratic freedoms. However, authoritarian governments have the latitude to abuse their power, and citizens' rights and welfare may be trivialized and deprioritized in favor of leaders' personal ambitions. The difference in the three countries' political systems has resulted in variations in their national pandemic responses. Compared to China's lockdowns, mandatory quarantine, and stay-at-home orders, Japan and South Korea mitigated the negative effects of the pandemic with a more humanitarian and democratic approach. Hence, as a democratic alternative to China's authoritarian approach, the Japanese and South Korean COVID-19 emergency management models provided valuable examples of how democracies can mitigate the ramifications of crises at a minimal cost to individual freedoms and inconvenience in citizens' daily lives (Kim, M. et al., 2020).

As previously mentioned, China, Japan, and South Korea not only share common characteristics but also differ in several respects. A comparison of them can offer valuable insights into the evolving state-society relations in East Asia. A successful strategy to handle the pandemic does not depend merely on the state's domination and control; citizens' cooperation and voluntary support are indispensable (Yan et al., 2020). Public opinion in China, Japan, and South Korea has shown how the COVID-19 pandemic has affected people's lives, and it provides vivid evidence of state-society relations in the three East Asian countries.

This book is based on the findings of a collaborative social survey conducted in China, Japan, and South Korea. At the research design stage, four social science researchers from China, Japan, and South Korea created an English questionnaire, which was translated into the three countries' local language. In all three countries, data collection was conducted through web-based nationwide sampling. The survey was administered in China from January 10, 2022, to January 20, 2022, and in Japan and South Korea between February 18, 2022, and March 3, 2022. All surveys adhered to the stratified quota sampling method. To increase the samples' representativeness, the sampling plan defined the subject quota by age group, gender, education, and area of residence. Given that the overall population composition differs across the three countries, the quota of demographic factors differed for each local survey. Respondent selection followed the quota, and we finally obtained 1,000 samples from each country. In the Chinese sample, respondents were aged 18 to 68 years, and men and women each accounted for 50%. In the Japanese sample, respondents were aged 18 to 79 years, and females and males accounted for 50.5%

and 49.5%, respectively. In the South Korean sample, respondents were aged 18 to 79 years, and women and men accounted for 49.3% and 50.7%, respectively.

Central Themes and Organization

This book provides insights into three East Asian countries' state-society relations amid the COVID-19 pandemic. Part I scrutinizes the dynamics of the state-society relationships in each country, offering details pertaining to trends of change in this relationship in the individual countries during the COVID-19 pandemic. Part II compares citizens' attitudes toward individual freedom, the state's anti-pandemic policies, vaccine hesitancy, and income redistribution policies across the three counties. Part III transcends national boundaries and focuses on citizens' evaluations of their domestic and neighboring countries' pandemic response.

Chapter 1 reviews the evolution of the COVID-19 pandemic and the government's response in China, Japan, and South Korea. These three governments adopted different countermeasures to control and prevent the spread of the virus, and the citizens of each country had different responses to their government's policies. The COVID-19 pandemic has reshaped state-society relations whereby governments have expanded their power and civil society has assisted government in this public health crisis. Citizens in these three countries showed high levels of compliance with their governments' anti-COVID-19 policies. This chapter further explains the theoretical importance of comparative studies of China, Japan, and South Korea and introduces datasets, methods of survey, and the book's central themes.

Chapter 2 provides an overview of the measures implemented in Japan to combat the COVID-19 pandemic. Japan's measures, which have been characterized as relatively soft, did not involve lockdowns or other restrictions on citizens' activities, instead relying on voluntary restraint. Rather than conducting widespread testing, the policy focused on dealing with individuals who displayed symptoms due to insufficient medical resources and digital capacity. This approach has been referred to as the "Japanese model."

Chapter 3 aims to shed new light on Korean society and politics during the COVID-19 pandemic. It examines why the early success of the Moon Jae-in government in combating COVID-19 did not lead to long-term political success. To address this question, this chapter focuses on government trust and its changes. There was a political paradox in Korea's success against COVID-19: The early success reduced public concerns and fear, causing Korean citizens to shift their focus to real estate and the economy. Negative performance evaluations on these two issues caused a decline in government trust from which the Moon Jae-in government could not recover. These results have important implications for Korean politics and society.

Chapter 4 analyzes Chinese citizens' anti-COVID-19 policy preferences, their willingness to comply with state policy, and attitudes toward the state's role in the economy. Since the initial outbreak of COVID-19, Chinese citizens have struggled for their lives. The government implemented stringent measures, including lockdowns and extended quarantine, and promoted a large-scale vaccination campaign. The voices of Chinese citizens provide important insights into the characteristics and sustainability of China's strategies for tackling COVID-19.

Chapter 5 provides a comparative analysis of the assessments made by citizens regarding the measures taken in response to COVID-19 in China, Japan, and South Korea with a particular focus on the impact of Asian values. The findings revealed that, initially, all three countries prioritized the prevention of infection over economic recovery, leading them to accept state intervention that restricted their freedom. Moreover, many COVID-19 measures and economic aid were widely supported as they aligned with Asian values. This was especially true in China, an authoritarian regime, where the influence of Asian values was more pronounced. There are no substantial discernible differences between Japan and South Korea. It is evident that the social hierarchies and group primacy that are prevalent in East Asian societies have contributed to the acceptance of state intervention in the region, which can be observed in the success of COVID-19 measures.

Chapter 6 examines how values prioritizing the group over the individual influence East Asian people's attitudes toward government economic relief during the COVID-19 pandemic. This chapter reveals that individuals who hold values emphasizing compliance with social norms and intolerance of deviant behavior from social norms are more likely to support economic relief measures across all three countries. This tendency is similar across the three countries, regardless of the differences in political regimes and specific COVID-19 measures. The conclusion enhances our understanding of East Asian countries' relative success in mitigating COVID-19 damage, suggesting that collectivist values may have facilitated not only people's compliance with behavioral restrictions but also their approval of economic support measures.

Chapter 7 addresses how perceptions of the role of luck influence people's attitudes toward economic relief policies during the COVID-19 pandemic in China, Japan, and South Korea. The results of our analyses of survey data from the three East Asian countries show that Japanese and Koreans who believe that luck affects people's achievement tend to have positive attitudes toward orthodox redistribution, which existing studies have found for Westerners. However, Chinese, Japanese, and Korean people who consider the economic damage caused by the pandemic to be due to bad luck are less likely to have positive attitudes toward economic support policies during the pandemic. These results imply that the pandemic has not changed people's expectations about the role of the state. Hence, the expansion of the state's economic role is unlikely to materialize.

Chapter 8 compares how East Asian citizens evaluated the COVID-19 governance systems that arose in China, Japan, and South Korea as a response to the pandemic's global spread. Beginning in 2020, the world was astounded to witness how the Western liberal democratic system—long thought to be the most developed political system—clearly displayed its own incapacity and inefficiency when confronted with the COVID-19 challenge. In contrast, East Asian countries routinely received excellent marks for their performance in the ratings of COVID-19 governance. In light of this broader context, this chapter retains a global perspective on East Asia while concentrating on China, Japan, and Korea to determine how the citizens of the three countries perceive their own nation's COVID-19 governance and those of other East Asian countries.

Chapter 9 compares Chinese, Japanese, and Korean citizens' perceptions of their countries' responses to the pandemic. It also analyzes how they view their counterpart countries' performance in tackling the pandemic. Information plays a critical role in shaping public opinion; hence, this chapter explains the variations in the evaluations of these countries' responses to the pandemic through information. This reveals the relationship between access to information and approval of the country's pandemic response in China, Japan, and South Korea. The results showed similarities and differences between the three countries.

References

Anderson, Roy M., Hans Heesterbeek, Don Klinkenberg, and T. Déirdre Hollingsworth. 2020. How will country-based mitigation measures influence the course of the COVID-19 epidemic? *Lancet* 395(10228): 931–934.

Cai, Qihai, Aya Okada, Bok Gyo Jeong, and Sung-Ju Kim. 2021. Civil society responses to the COVID-19 pandemic. *China Review* 21(1): 107–138.

CGTN. 2020. Wuhan police apologize for reprimanding doctor who sounded early alarm on COVID-19. March 19, 2020. https://news.cgtn.com/news/2020-03-19/Admonition-letter-to-Dr-Li-Wenliang-improper-investigation-OZvG7i94Fa/index.html

Chen, Haiqian, Leiyu Shi, Yuyao Zhang, Xiaohan Wang, and Gang Sun. 2021. A cross-country core strategy comparison in China, Japan, Singapore and South Korea during the early COVID-19 pandemic. *Globalization and Health* 17: 22.

Chen, Sylvia Xiaohua, Ben C. P. Lam, James H. Liu, Hoon-Seok Choi, Emiko Kashima, and Allan B. I. Bernardo. 2021. Effects of containment and closure policies on controlling the COVID-19 pandemic in East Asia. *Asian Journal of Social Psychology* 24: 42–47.

Chiavacci, David and Julia Obinger. 2018. Towards a new protest cycle in contemporary Japan? In David Chiavacci and Julia Obinger (eds.), *Social Movements and Political Activism in Contemporary Japan: Re-emerging from Invisibility*. London: Routledge, pp. 1–23.

Cho, Youngho, Mi-son Kim, and Yong Cheol Kim. 2019. Cultural foundation of contentious democracy in South Korea: What democracy do Korean citizens prefer? *Asian Survey* 59(2): 272–294.

Choi, Yon Jung. 2020. The power of collaborative governance: The case of South Korea responding to COVID-19 pandemic. *World Med Health Policy* 12(4): 430–442.

Druckman, Daniel. 1994. Nationalism, patriotism, and group loyalty: A social psychological perspective. *Mershon International Studies Review* 38: 43–68.

Du, Zhanwei, Lin Wang, Simon Cauchemez, Xiaoke Xu, Xianwen Wang, Benjamin J. Cowling, and Lauren Ancel Meyers. 2020. Risk for transportation of 2019 novel coronavirus disease from Wuhan to other cities in China. *Emerging Infectious Diseases* 26(5): 1049–1052.

Falch, Daniel and Christopher D. Hammond. 2020. Social activism and "spaces of autonomy" in the context of Japan: An analysis of the student movement known as SEALDs. *Globalisation, Societies and Education* 18(4): 435–448.

Fiori, Antonio and Sunhyuk Kim. 2018. Civil society and democracy in South Korea: A reassessment. In Youngmi Kim (ed.), *Korea's Quest for Economic Democratization*. New York: Palgrave Macmillan, pp. 141–170.

Guan, Yue, Lei Guang, Lianjiang Li, and Yanchuan Liu. 2024. The rally effect of the COVID-19 pandemic and the White Paper Movement in China. *Journal of Contemporary China*, DOI: 10.1080/10670564.2024.2356863.

Haggard, Stephan. 2018. *Developmental States. Elements in the Politics of Development.* Cambridge: Cambridge University Press.

Hasegawa, Kōichi. 2018. Continuities and discontinuities of Japan's political activism before and after the Fukushima disaster. In David Chiavacci and Julia Obinger (eds.), *Social Movements and Political Activism in Contemporary Japan: Re-emerging from Invisibility*. London: Routledge, pp. 115–136.

Hsu, Jennifer Y. J. and Reza Hasmath. 2014. The local corporatist state and NGO relations in China. *Journal of Contemporary China* 23(87): 516–534.

Ikeda, Ken'ichi. 2022. *Contemporary Japanese Politics and Anxiety over Governance.* London: Routledge.

Im, Tobin. 2020. COVID-19 national report on South Korea: Competitive bureaucratic leadership taking lessons from prior experiences. In Paul Joyce, Fabienne Maron, and Purshottama Sivanarain Reddy (eds.), *Good Public Governance in a Global Pandemic.* Brussels: The International Institute of Administrative Sciences, pp. 221–230.

Inoue, Hajime. 2020. Japanese strategy to COVID-19: How does it work? *Global Health & Medicine* 2(2): 131–132.

Jee, Youngmee. 2020. Making sense of South Korea's response to COVID-19. In Paul Joyce, Fabienne Maron, and Purshottama Sivanarain Reddy (eds.), *Good Public Governance in a Global Pandemic.* Brussels: The International Institute of Administrative Sciences, pp. 85–87.

Jia, Ziyu, Shijia Xu, Zican Zhang, Zhengyu Cheng, Haoqing Han, Haoxiang Xu, Mingtian Wang, Hong Zhang, Yi Zhou, and Zhengxu Zhou. 2021. Association between mental health and community support in lockdown communities during the COVID-19 pandemic: Evidence from rural China. *Journal of Rural Studies* 82: 87–97.

Jung, Gyuwon, Hyunsoo Lee, Auk Kim, and Uichin Lee. 2020. Too much information: Assessing privacy risks of contact trace data disclosure on people with COVID-19 in South Korea. *Frontiers in Public Health* 8: 305.

Kang, Xiaoguang and Han Heng. 2008. Graduated Controls: The State-Society Relationship in Contemporary China. *Modern China* 34(1): 36–55.Kim, Hyuk-Rae. 2000. The state and civil society in transition: The role of non-governmental organizations in South Korea. *The Pacific Review* 13(4): 595–613.

Kim, Min-Hyu, Wonhyuk Cho, Hemin Choi, and Joon-Young Hur. 2020. Assessing the South Korean model of emergency management during the COVID-19 pandemic. *Asian Studies Review* 44(4): 567–578.

Kim, Sungjoong, Sung Kyum Cho, and Sarah Prusoff LoCascio. 2020. The role of media use and emotions in risk perception and preventive behaviors related to COVID-19 in South Korea. *Asian Journal for Public Opinion Research* 8(3): 297–323.

Kim, Sunhyuk. 2000. *The Politics of Democratization in Korea: The Role of Civil Society.* Pittsburgh: University of Pittsburgh Press.

Kim, Sunhyuk and Jong-Ho Jeong. 2017. Historical development of civil society in Korea since 1987. *Journal of International and Area Studies* 24(2): 1–14.

Kim, Uichol, Harry C. Triandis, Cigdem Kagitcibasi, Sang-Chin Choi, and Gene Yoon. 1994. *Individualism and Collectivism: Theory, Method, and Applications*. Thousand Oaks, CA: Sage.

Kim, Woojin Tae Yong Jung, Susann Roth, Woochong Um, and Changsoo Kim. 2021. Management of the COVID-19 pandemic in the Republic of Korea from the perspective of governance and public-private partnership. *Yonsei Medical Journal* 62(9): 777–791.

Kingston, Jeff. 2015. SEALDs: Students slam Abe's assault on Japan's constitution. *The Asia-Pacific Journal* 13(36): 1–9.

Kupferschmidt, Kai and Jon Cohen. 2020. Can China's COVID-19 strategy work elsewhere? *Science* 367(6482): 1061–1062.

Kyriacou, Andreas P. 2016. Individualism–collectivism, governance and economic development. *European Journal of Political Economy* 42: 91–104.

Lee, Daejoong, Kyungmoo Heo, Yongseok Seo. 2020. COVID-19 in South Korea: Lessons for developing countries. *World Development* 135: 105057.

Lee, Sabinne, Changho Hwang, and M. Jae Moon. 2020. Policy learning and crisis policy-making: Quadruple-loop learning and COVID-19 responses in South Korea. *Policy and Society* 39(3): 363–381.

Lu, Ning, Kai-Wen Cheng, Nafees Qamar, Kuo-Cherh Huang, and James A Johnson. 2020. Weathering COVID-19 storm: Successful control measures of five Asian countries. *American Journal of Infection Control* 48(7): 851–852.

Ma, Xiaohua. 2020. From no evidence of human-to-human transmission to existence of human-to-human transmission. Yicai, January 21, 2020. www.yicai.com/news/100476157.html. (in Chinese)

Machimura, Takashi and Keiichi Satoh (eds.). 2016. *Citizens Taking Action for a Nuclear Free Society: A Sociology of Social Movements after 3.11*. Tokyo: Shinyosha. (in Japanese)

Moon, M. Jae. 2020. Fighting COVID-19 with agility, transparency, and participation: Wicked policy problems and new governance challenges. *Public Administration Review* 80(4): 651–656.

Moon, M. Jae, Kohei Suzuki, Tae In Park, and Kentaro Sakuwa. 2021. A comparative study of COVID-19 responses in South Korea and Japan: Political nexus triad and policy responses. *International Review of Administrative Sciences* 87(3): 651–671.

Ogawa, Akihiro. 2004. Invited by the state: Institutionalizing volunteer subjectivity in contemporary Japan. *Asian Anthropology* 3(1): 71–96.

Ogawa, Akihiro. 2019. Civil society: Past, present, and future. In Jeff Kingston (ed.), *Critical Issues in Contemporary Japan* (2nd). London: Routledge, pp. 47–58.

Ogawa, Akihiro. 2021. Civil society in Japan. In Robert Pekkanen and Saadia Pekkanen (eds.), *Oxford Handbook of Japanese Politics*. New York: Oxford University Press, pp. 299–316.

Oguma, Eiji. 2016. A new wave against the rock: New social movements in Japan since the Fukushima nuclear meltdown. *The Asia-Pacific Journal Japan Focus* 14(13-2): 1–39.

Oh, Jennifer S. 2012. Strong state and strong civil society in contemporary South Korea: Challenges to democratic governance. *Asian Survey* 52(3): 528–549.

Park, Sangchul, Gina Jeehyun Choi, and Haksoo Ko. 2020. Information technology-based tracing strategy in response to COVID-19 in South Korea: Privacy controversies. *Journal of American Medical Association* 323(21): 2129–2130.

Pekkanen, Robert. 2006. *Japan's Dual Civil Society: Members without Advocates*. Stanford, CA: Stanford University Press.

Salamon, Lester M. and S. Wojciech Sokolowski. 2004. *Global Civil Society: Dimensions of the Nonprofit Sector*. Boulder, CO: Kumarian Press.

Shaw, Rajib, Yong-kyun Kim, and Jinling Hua. 2020. Governance, technology and citizen behavior in pandemic: Lessons from COVID-19 in East Asia. *Progress in Disaster Science* 6: 100090.

Shimizu, Kazuki and Masashi Negita. 2020. Lessons learned from Japan's response to the first wave of COVID-19: A content analysis. *Healthcare* 8: 426.

Shimizu, Kazuki, George Wharton, Haruka Sakamoto, and Elias Mossialos. 2020. Resurgence of covid-19 in Japan. *British Medical Journal* 370: m3221.

Shin, Doh Chull. 2012. *Confucianism and Democratization in East Asia*. New York: Cambridge University Press.

Shiroyama, Hideaki. 2020. Japan's response to the COVID-19. In Paul Joyce, Fabienne Maron, and Purshottama Sivanarain Reddy (eds.), *Good Public Governance in a Global Pandemic*. Brussels: The International Institute of Administrative Sciences, pp. 195–204.

Tsuji, Yuichiro. 2022. Political power and the limits of academic freedom in Japan in the era of Covid-19. *Australian Journal of Asian Law* 22(2): 117–130.

Tu, Wei-ming. 1996. *Confucian Traditions in East Asian Modernity: Moral Education and Economic Culture in Japan and the Four Mini-Dragons*. Cambridge, MA: Harvard University Press.

Wang, Chen, Peter W. Horby, Frederick G. Hayden, and George F. Gao. 2020. A novel coronavirus outbreak of global health concern. *Lancet* 395: 470–473.

Wang, Manchuan. 2020. Responses of the central government of China to COVID-19 pandemic: Major decisions and lessons. In Paul Joyce, Fabienne Maron, and Purshottama Sivanarain Reddy (eds.), *Good Public Governance in a Global Pandemic*. Brussels: The International Institute of Administrative Sciences, pp. 161–170.

WHO. 2022. Coronavirus disease (COVID-19) Pandemic. Available at https://covid19.who.int/.

Woo-Cumings, Meredith. 1999. *The Developmental State*. Ithaca, NY: Cornell University Press.

Woods, Eric Taylor, Robert Schertzer, Liah Greenfeld, Chris Hughes, and Cynthia Miller-Idriss. 2020. COVID-19, nationalism, and the politics of crisis: A scholarly exchange. *Nations and Nationalism* 26(4): 807–825.

Wright, James. 2021. Overcoming political distrust: The role of "self-restraint" in Japan's public health response to COVID-19. *Japan Forum* 33(4): 453–475.

Wu, Fang, Qi Hu, Chenming Zhu, HaitaoWang, Qian Yu, and Huaping Sun. 2021. New structural economic analysis of anti-COVID-19 pandemic model of BEST region. *International Journal of Environmental Research and Public Health* 18: 7822.

Yan, Bo, Xiaomin Zhang, Long Wu, Heng Zhu, and Bin Chen. 2020. Why do countries respond differently to COVID-19? A comparative study of Sweden, China, France, and Japan. *American Review of Public Administration* 50(6-7): 762–769.

Zeng, Qingjie. 2024. Strict COVID-19 lockdown and popular regime support in China. *Democratization* 31(7): 1373–1396.

Zhai, Yida. 2022. Values change and support for democracy in East Asia. *Social Indicators Research* 160(1): 179–198.

Zhai, Yida. 2023. The politics of COVID-19: Political logic of China's Zero-COVID policy. *Journal of Contemporary Asia* 53(5): 869–886.

Zhai, Yida. 2024. Outgroup threat, ideology, and favorable evaluations of the government's responses to COVID-19. *Current Psychology* 43: 13110–13119.

Zhai, Yida and Guanghua Han. 2024. Lockdown, information quality, and political trust: An empirical study of the Shanghai lockdown under COVID-19. *International Review of Administrative Sciences* 90(1): 132–148.

Zhang, Wanqing. 2020. Human transmission of Wuhan pneumonia "cannot be ruled out." *Sixth Tone*, Jan 15, 2020. www.sixthtone.com/news/1005079/human-transmission-of-wuhan-pneumonia-cannot-be-ruled-out

Zhao, Shilei and Hua Chen. 2020. Modeling the epidemic dynamics and control of COVID-19 outbreak in China. *Quantitative Biology* 8(1): 11–19.

Part I

Focus on Changes in State-Society Relations in Japan, South Korea, and China

2 Review of Japan's Corona Policy

Interaction between the Government and Citizens

Hidehiro Yamamoto

Introduction

This chapter will provide a summary of Japan's COVID-19 control measures. While Japan, like Korea and China, has successfully controlled the number of cases and deaths related to COVID-19, there are differences in the approach taken by each country.

Japan's measures, which have been characterized as relatively soft (Shiroyama, 2020; Asia Pacific Initiative, 2020), did not involve lockdowns or other restrictions on citizens' activities, instead relying on voluntary restraint. Rather than conducting widespread infection testing, the policy focused on dealing with individuals who displayed symptoms. This approach has been referred to as the "Japanese model" (Asia Pacific Initiative, 2020). Additionally, a large financial outlay was provided to support the economy during the pandemic. Throughout the COVID-19 crisis, local governments played an active role in responding to the situation. Therefore, this chapter will also examine the policy process from the perspective of the relationship between the central and local governments.

In addition, this chapter examine the impact of COVID-19 on the lives of citizens using a questionnaire survey conducted independently in Japan in January 2021; this is followed by an evaluation of policy and political actors.

Political Situations in Japan

Prior to assessing the measures implemented in response to the COVID-19 pandemic, it is essential to analyze Japan's political climate. Since the early 1990s, the country has embarked on a series of political reforms, encompassing electoral, administrative, and decentralization measures. The most significant of these reforms was the introduction of a dual electoral system, comprising single-seat constituencies and proportional representation, in the House of Representatives elections. The implementation of this system was anticipated to reduce the number of effective political parties and facilitate the emergence of a two-party dominant system (Sasaki, 1999). The rationale behind such reform was to break up the prolonged one-party-dominated political landscape, characterized by the Liberal Democratic Party (LDP) (Machidori, 2020). Furthermore, when only one seat is up

DOI: 10.4324/9781003495239-3

for grabs in an election, the process of selecting a candidate becomes of paramount importance for each political party. This has resulted in a centralization of power within the party leadership (Machidori, 2020; Takenaka, 2017, 2019).

The significant impact on Japan's administrative system has been the fortification of cabinet functions through reforms. This has led to the establishment of a decision-making system wherein authority is centralized in the hands of the prime minister, often referred to as "prime ministerial leadership (*shusho shihai*)." The previous policy formation process, which was characterized by coordination between the ruling LDP, the bureaucracy, and interest groups, has now transitioned to a hierarchical approach dictated by the prime minister (Machidori, 2012, 2020; Takenaka, 2017, 2019).

Since the late 1990s, major changes have been made to the electoral system in Japan, resulting in the strengthening of the largest opposition parties, such as the Democratic Party of Japan (DPJ) and the emergence of a two-party system comprising the LDP and the DPJ. This shift ultimately led to a change in government in 2009, when the coalition of the LDP and Komeito was replaced by a government led by the DPJ. During its time in power, the DPJ focused on reforms, such as promoting political leadership, but it lost public support due to its poor handling of the Great East Japan Earthquake and the Fukushima nuclear accident, as well as growing internal conflicts within the party.

Following the 2012 general election, a coalition government comprising the LDP and the Komeito party was reestablished. Under the administration of Shinzo Abe, the LDP achieved victory in six national elections for both the lower and upper houses, enabling it to exercise stable parliamentary power. Conversely, the DPJ suffered defeat and subsequently fragmented into multiple factions, failing to coalesce into a single formidable force. During this time, the Japan Restoration Association (*Nihon ishin no kai. Ishin*) emerged, but it failed to rival the LDP in terms of competitive strength. Furthermore, Ishin shared a conservative ideological stance similar to that of the LDP, precluding the formation of an opposing political axis.

The second Abe Administration was known for its centralized system of authority, which allowed for policy decisions to be made in a top-down fashion under the leadership of the prime minister and the prime minister's office (Nakakita, 2022). This approach led to a decrease in the influence of other ruling party legislators, bureaucrats, and interest groups (Takenaka, 2017).

The centerpiece of the Abe administration was Abenomics—a comprehensive economic policy aimed at reviving the Japanese economy. The policy was based on three key principles: significant monetary easing, aggressive fiscal stimulus, and structural reforms designed to encourage private sector investment. Additionally, the government implemented policies to support women and labor, as part of its broader objective to create a more active society and reform the workplace.

In the realm of foreign policy, Japan demonstrated an assertive approach to its national security. In addition to establishing the National Security Council, it enacted the Peace and Security Legislation in 2015, which included the right to exercise collective self-defense, despite widespread protests. Around this time, Japan achieved notable diplomatic successes, such as the Prime Minister's Statement on the 70th anniversary of the end of World War II, a significant agreement on the TPP negotiations, and the Japan-Korea Comfort Women Agreement. Moreover, Abe advocated for constitutional reform, although his efforts to bring it about were unsuccessful. Abe's political ideology was characterized by a strong nationalistic orientation, and he sought a governance model that emphasized strong leadership.

During the latter part of his administration, Abe faced challenges in fully promoting his policies due to a series of political scandals involving himself. The concluding phase of his tenure was predominantly focused on implementing measures in response to the COVID-19 pandemic.

The Yoshihide Suga Administration, which came into power in September 2020 following the Abe Administration, pursued Abe's policies while also attempting to introduce new policies such as digitalization and carbon neutrality. However, due to the recurring COVID-19 outbreaks, the government's focus shifted entirely toward COVID-19 measures during its tenure. Despite this, Suga managed to host the Tokyo Olympic and Paralympic Games, which had been postponed from the previous year. The following Fumio Kishida Administration advovated for "new capitalism" and implemented an economic growth strategy aimed at addressing distributional and income inequality issues.

History of COVID-19 Measures in Japan[1]

Central Government COVID-19 Measures and Society

In January 2020, the initial case of COVID-19 in Japan was reported. Following the outbreak in Wuhan, China, the Japanese government initiated efforts to repatriate its citizens residing in the affected area via chartered aircraft. Shortly thereafter, border control measures were implemented, including entry restrictions and quarantine systems, in countries where the virus had spread. On January 30, the government established "the Headquarters for New Coronavirus Control (*Shingata Korona Uirusu Kansensho Taisaku Honbu*)." On February 1, COVID-19 was classed as a "designated infectious disease (*Shitei Kansen Sho*)."

In February, the outbreak on the Diamond Princess, a cruise ship docked in the port of Yokohama, garnered significant attention. Due to the absence of medical facilities in Japan capable of quarantining and accommodating more than 3,000 crew members and passengers, the ship was quarantined and isolated for approximately two weeks. The Japanese government faced substantial criticism for its inadequate response to this unprecedented situation (Nihon Keizai Shimbun, February 12, 2022).

The number of individuals contracting the virus through unidentified means rose in the city from February to March, and, consequently, the government's approach transitioned from restricting entry to emphasizing domestic infection control measures (Shaw et al., 2020). Despite the growing number of infected individuals, the local public health centers, which were the first to receive consultation on the infection, were unable to keep pace. Additionally, the legal framework restricted the number of designated medical institutions that could accept patients with the virus, making it difficult to secure hospital beds. The operations of these medical institutions were strained, resulting in a state of medical crisis. For this reason, the Japanese government adopted measures to test only those people suspected of being infected. This was different from the situation in Korea and China, where PCR testing was expanded to prevent quarantine.

The "Novel Coronavirus Expert Meeting (*Shingata Korona Uirusu Kansensho Taisaku Senmonka Kaigi*)," a gathering of experts in infectious diseases, was established to provide advice from a medical perspective.[2] The goal, in the meeting's view, was to control the speed of the spread of the infection and to reduce the incidence of severe cases and deaths as much as possible, given the limitations of medical resources.[3]

The experts highlighted the necessity of suppressing clusters containing infected individuals, which was echoed in the government's "Basic Policy on Countermeasures against Infectious Diseases (*Kansensho Taisaku no Kihon Hoshin*)." The government specified three conditions under which clusters are most likely to emerge: enclosed spaces (*Mippei*), crowded areas (*Misshu*), and settings involving close contact (*Missetsu*), collectively referred to as the "*San Mitsu*" in Japanese, which translates to "3C" in English. In response, the government implemented measures to prevent these conditions from occurring.

In March, the Abe Administration amended the existing "Law Concerning Special Measures Against Novel Influenza (*Shingata Infuruenza Tou Taisaku Tokubetsu Sochi Hou*)" so that it could be applied to COVID-19. Under the revised law, prefectural governors in the affected areas could ask residents to refrain from leaving their homes and cooperate in other ways necessary to prevent the spread of the infection. The governors could also request the closure of schools and restaurants, as well as the placement of restrictions on the use of department stores, movie theaters, and other facilities that attract a large number of people. Furthermore, they could use land or buildings without the owner's consent to establish temporary medical facilities or expropriate medical supplies if necessary.

The emergency declaration was officially proclaimed for Tokyo, Kanagawa, Saitama, Chiba, Osaka, Hyogo, and Fukuoka on April 7, ultimately encompassing the entire nation on April 16. The declaration exceeded its initial timeline, lasting until the end of May. Although closures and restrictions on events were suggested, they were not mandatory, and penalties were rarely imposed. Japan's legal framework did not permit the implementation of stringent measures to combat COVID-19.

Therefore, Japan's countermeasures depended on its citizens. Although hoarding panic broke out in the early days when masks and other hygiene products were scarce, citizens also engaged in self-limiting social activities (*jishuku*) without much opposition to the government measures. Work arrangements that took advantage of an online presence, such as telecommuting, also became widespread. Also observed was certain over-adaptive behavior, termed "self-restraint police (*jishuku keisatsu*)," such as blaming those not wearing masks or others from outside the area (Matsubara 2021).

The government's response to the ongoing crisis includes several noteworthy points. Firstly, on March 24, 2020, the decision was made to postpone the Tokyo Olympics and Paralympics Games for one year. Although the possibility of hosting the event was explored, it was ultimately decided to abandon the idea due to the significant health risks posed to athletes, officials, and spectators, as well as the restrictions on importing in various countries and the growing criticism of the event.

In response to the surge in demand for masks, the government implemented a policy of distributing two cloth masks to each household. Despite the significant financial investment required, this initiative was not met with public approval (Asahi Shimbun, April 21, 2020) and was ridiculed by the public, who referred to it as the "*Abenomask*" in reference to the then prime minister Abe.

Economic support to maintain employment, continue business operations, support livelihoods, and restore economic activity was also important. The special fixed benefit (*tokubetsu teigaku kyofukin*) in April 2020, which provided a flat amount of 100,000 yen per person regardless of the level of economic loss or poverty, was noteworthy. Additionally, continuous livelihood compensation was provided by the government and local governments to companies and people who were forced to close their businesses.

Following the summer of 2020, when the outbreak had subsided, the Japanese government introduced a campaign known as GO TO Travel and GO TO Eat with the aim of supporting the tourism and restaurant sectors, which had been particularly affected, and stimulating overall economic activity. To achieve this objective, the government provided subsidies to reduce the cost of travel and dining. However, the recurring outbreak of the disease in November necessitated the cancelation of several campaigns, resulting in limited success for the initiative.

The Japanese government allocated significant funds toward a range of measures aimed at combating COVID-19, including the passage of three unprecedented supplementary budgets in FY2020 (Yomiuri Shimbun Tokyo Head Office, Research Division 2022). According to the International Monetary Fund's (IMF) financial report, Japan ranked second after the United States in terms of fiscal spending at the end of 2020 (Sankei Shimbun, January 29, 2021), despite having a relatively small number of infected individuals and deaths compared to other developed countries.

The Suga Administration, which came into power in September 2020, carried on with the policies of the previous Abe Administration. The Suga Administration aimed to promote initiatives such as digitalization and carbon neutrality. However, throughout its tenure, there were recurring waves of COVID-19 infection: the third wave from November 2020 to the end of February 2021, the fourth wave from the end of March to June, and the fifth wave from July to September. These waves led to the implementation of emergency measures and the issuance of priority measures to curb the spread of the virus in specific regions. Despite the ongoing state of emergency, the Tokyo Olympics and Paralympic Games, which had been postponed the previous year, were held in July.

The COVID-19 response plan of the Suga Administration emphasized the importance of vaccination. Japan was initially slow in acquiring vaccines and had low vaccination rates. The appointment of a vaccine minister expedited preparations. The government committed to vaccinating all elderly individuals who desired it by the end of July, and it urged each municipality to do the same. By the end of October 2009, 71.2% of the entire population had received two vaccinations, and among the elderly, the figure exceeded 90% (Mainichi Shimbun, October 30, 2021).

However, the prevalence of the ailment could not be curtailed, which impacted the cabinet's approval rating and resulted in the unpopularity of the Suga Administration. Subsequently, Suga was compelled to resign in September, paving the way for the Kishida Administration. Following its victory in the October Lower House election, the Kishida Administration introduced supportive benefits for households with children as a response to COVID-19.[4]

Subsequently, the number of cases surged during the sixth wave from January to March 2010, the seventh wave from July to September 2010, and the eighth wave from January to March 2011. However, the rates of severe illness and mortality diminished. As a result, a policy to revert to normalcy was proposed, and in May 2023 the decision was taken to reclassify COVID-19 from an infectious disease presenting a high risk of severe illness to a status equal to that of seasonal influenza. Subsequently, no emergency declarations or requests for closures were put forth. Recommendations for wearing masks and limitations on large-scale events also have been lifted.

Central-Local Government Relationships Regarding COVID-19 Measures

In the central government, decisions regarding infection control measures were made in a top-down fashion under a power structure headed by the prime minister. For instance, the Prime Minister's Office was responsible for determining measures such as the closure of public schools and the distribution of cloth masks to each household, as well as the GO TO Campaign (Takenaka, 2021).

However, the law also provided for prefectural authorities to implement policies; thus, local governments were proactive in their efforts. For instance, Hokkaido, where the outbreak began early, issued a state of emergency and closed elementary and junior high schools. Osaka also took preemptive measures ahead of the central government, such as securing hospital beds and establishing objective numerical criteria for lifting the state of emergency declaration. Governors who took these initiatives received high accolades; consequently, COVID-19 created an avenue for local governments to implement their own measures, thereby fostering a competitive environment for performance among local governments (Sunahara, 2020).

Conflicts between the central and local governments have also been observed (Shiroyama,2020; Takenaka, 2021). A notable instance was the clash between the central government and the Tokyo Metropolitan Government regarding the declaration of a state of emergency. Tokyo governor Yuriko Koike aimed to implement a more extensive shutdown of the central government after the state of emergency. However, the government was apprehensive about the economic repercussions and did not envision an immediate closure. Consequently, the Tokyo Metropolitan

Government requested closures, albeit with a reduced scope of industries covered, and other prefectures followed suit. Osaka prefecture's decision to lift its emergency declaration by presenting quantifiable standards was met with criticism from the central government. As a result, while prefectures concentrated on controlling the spread of infection, the central government sometimes adopted a passive stance due to concerns about its negative economic impact (Takenaka, 2021).

Conversely, the central government aimed to implement economic support measures, such as promoting tourism through "GO TO Travel" initiatives; however, the governors argued that such measures were premature (Sankei Shimbun, July 17, 2020), and the prefectures responded in the opposite manner, urging self-restraint in travel to curb the spread of infection (Takenaka, 2021). In another case, while the central government demonstrated robust support for the vaccination campaign and local governments backed the drive, instances emerged where the import and supply of vaccines failed to keep pace, creating associated challenges.

As previously discussed, in the context of COVID-19 measures, although the central government established the general policy framework, local governments were often authorized to implement specific policies within the legal system. Consequently, there arose instances where the central government's top-down policy formation and execution proved ineffective. The public also appreciated the governor's proactive approach in advancing ahead of the central government. Thus, COVID-19 may have transformed central-local government relations in Japan.

Characteristics of Japan's COVID-19 Measures

The following is a summary of the distinctive features of Japan's COVID-19 response measures. Initially, Japan adopted a voluntary approach, urging citizens to exercise restraint rather than imposing strict measures such as lockdowns. A significant number of people willingly complied with the government's request to avoid activities like community gatherings, leaving home, and eating out (Hanibuchi et al., 2021; Kashima and Zhang, 2021; Muto et al., 2020). Some individuals even went to the extent of condemning those who did not comply, and those persons could be referred to as the "self-restraint police (*Jishuku Keisatsu*)."

Despite this, the Japanese people had low confidence in their government (Taniguchi et al., 2022; Vardavas et al., 2021). This contrasted with their positive response to the government's request. It highlighted the critical role that trust in health professionals and the healthcare system played in shaping citizen behavior (Okada et al., 2022). However, other factors must be investigated further to provide a comprehensive understanding of Japan's COVID-19 response.

Second, and as previously stated, Japan did not carry out extensive PCR testing. This was due to insufficient medical resources and the need to allocate facilities, such as hospital beds, to symptomatic patients. Another factor contributing to Japan's insufficient inspections may be its failure to effectively employ digital technology. Korea and China made use of digital technology to monitor their citizens' behavior and actively promoted widespread testing and treatment (Moon et al., 2021; Shaw et al., 2020). Contrastingly, in Japan, the COVID-19

Contact-Confirming Application (COCOA) was developed, but it did not gain widespread usage. This was due to numerous issues with the application and the public's low level of trust.

Third, digitization of information sharing in Japan was not fully realized due to differences in laws and ordinances between the central government and individual local governments during the COVID-19 pandemic. To address this issue, a system called HER-SYS was introduced to share information about infected individuals. However, the system was not initially fully operational, and fax machines were used to transmit information in large municipalities such as Tokyo and Osaka. This was not only due to the rapid increase in the number of infected individuals but also because each municipality had established its own tallying system (Tokyo Shimbun, July 27, 2020).

Of course, the COVID-19 pandemic has brought about significant changes to Japanese lifestyles, with online meetings and online consumption becoming the norm. However, there was a noticeable delay in the administrative response to the pandemic.

COVID-19 and Citizens' Lives in Japan

Impact on Citizens' Lives

Prior to delving into the comparative analysis that is presented subsequently in this book, it is useful to examine the impact of COVID-19 on the lives of Japanese citizens, as well as the evaluations they have made regarding specific policies and political figures based on original data from Japan.

The data I used here differs from that of the other chapters in that it was collected solely in Japan during January 2021. The web survey was commissioned by the Japanese research company, Rakuten Insight, Inc., and targeted individuals aged 18 to 79 who resided throughout Japan among the company's registered monitors. In order to closely match the population composition, sex, age, and prefecture of residence were taken into account. It is important to note that January 2021 marked the peak of the third wave of the epidemic, and at that time the GO TO Campaign, a policy aimed at stimulating travel and eating out demand, and boosting the economy, was canceled under the Suga Administration.

Figure 2.1 illustrates the findings regarding the impact of COVID-19 on livelihoods. The survey inquired about the degree to which ten specific issues affected the respondents. The question employed a 6-point scale, with the option of "not concerned" included. The figure shows the percentages of responses where there was a concern. Results indicated that around 20% of the respondents were "significantly affected" by going out, acquiring masks, and interacting with others. In addition, over 70% stated that they were "affected" or "somewhat affected." It is not surprising that behavioral restrictions and routine infection prevention measures had the most widespread influence. However, 76% of the respondents were "not much affected,""little affected," or "not affected" with regard to the difficulty in handling information devices.

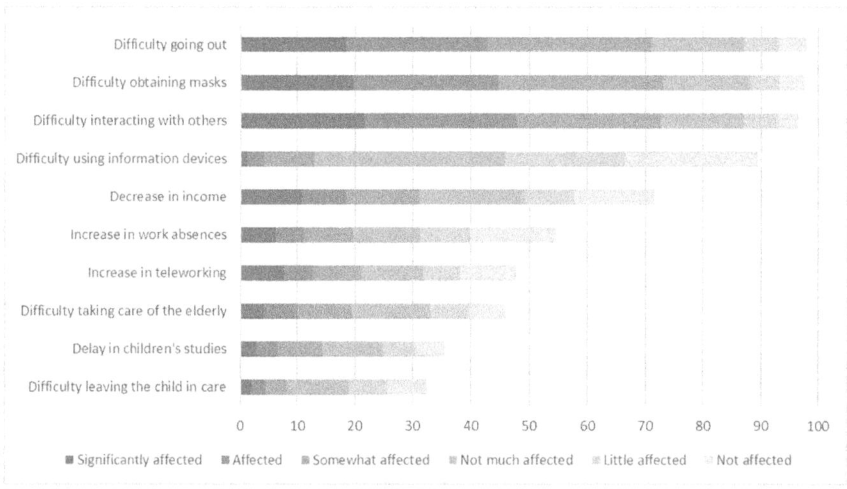

Figure 2.1 Impact of COVID-19 on livelihoods.

In response to the decrease in income, 31% of the population reported that it had impacted them to some degree (comprising "significantly affected,""affected," and "somewhat affected"). However, other issues were not of concern for more than 40% of the population. With regard to work, among those who were affected, 36% of respondents experienced an increase in work absences and 44% of those encountering an increase in teleworking reported being affected. Issues related to childcare and caregiving were less prevalent. Among those affected, 42% reported being impacted by taking care of the elderly, and 40% by delays in their children's studies. Leaving the child in care affected 25%. Across all the issues, there was a certain level of impact, but an unsubstantial number of people were affected.

Evaluation of Political Actors and Policy-making Process

Let us now examine the citizens' evaluation of the Japanese government's policies discussed in this chapter. Prior studies have shown that support for and compliance with COVID-19 measures depend on partisanship (Altiparmakis et al., 2021; Hata, 2024; Jørgensen et al., 2021; Yamamoto and Fujita, 2023). Therefore, we will review the results for supporters of the ruling parties, the LDP and Komeito, as well as supporters of other parties and those without a party preference.

Table 2.1 shows the means of the results when survey participants were asked about each measure on a 6-point scale; indeed, the statistical test assessed the difference in means between ruling party supporters and others. A higher value indicates a higher evaluation. On all measures, supporters of the ruling party were rated higher than the rest of the population. Supporters of the ruling party had a mean value generally around 4.0, above the midpoint of 3.5 on the 6-point scale. In contrast, the rest of the respondents were around 3.5, with no strong positive or negative attitudes.

Table 2.1 Evaluation of each COVID-19 measure: Mean comparison of ruling party supporters and others

	Ruling party supporters	*Others*	*t values*
State of emergency declaration	4.32	3.74	8.99**
Distribution of cloth masks	2.49	1.71	12.77**
Special fixed benefit	4.63	4.08	8.26**
Economic support for businesses	4.15	3.57	9.33**
Economic support for individuals	4.05	3.54	8.32**
Restrictions on immigration of Japanese nationals	4.18	3.68	7.54**
Restrictions on immigration of foreigners	4.09	3.60	6.70**
Request for voluntary restraint of movement	4.10	3.61	7.60**
Restrictions on holding events	4.17	3.72	6.82**
Requests for closure or reduced business hours	3.99	3.56	6.77**
School closings	3.84	3.34	8.02**
GO TO Travel	3.08	2.43	8.72**
GO TO Eat	3.05	2.44	8.37**
N	595	1406	

* $p < .05$, ** $p < .01$.

The highest-rated policy was the special benefit of 100,000 yen per person, with a score of 4.63 among supporters of the ruling party and 4.08 among others. However, the distribution of cloth masks, known as "*Abenomasks*," was not well-received, with a score of 2.49 among supporters of the ruling party and 1.71 among the rest. Additionally, the GO TO Travel and GO TO Eat campaigns, which aimed to help recover from economic damage, were rated poorly with a mean value of approximately 3.1 for ruling party supporters and 2.4 for others. This may be due to the controversy surrounding the campaign during the survey period, caused by the spread of the virus.

According to previous indications, the confidence of the Japanese public in the government's handling of COVID-19 measures was relatively low. Furthermore, the implementation of these measures was perceived as a struggle between the central government, which is becoming increasingly centralized under the leadership of the prime minister, and the prefectures, which possess the authority to implement the policy. The question remains, which of these two actors did citizens value more?

Table 2.2 displays the evaluation of each political actor in the COVID-19 measures. Means are denoted by whether or not they are supporters of the ruling party, and the results of the statistical tests are appended. The scores, which range from 1 to 6 on a scale (with higher scores indicating higher ratings), illustrate the public's assessment of the measures.

Supporters of the ruling parties (LDP and Komeito) gave higher ratings for the prime minister, central government ministries, and the ruling party, with a mean score of 3.5, approximately the midpoint of the 6-point scale. In contrast, the mean

Table 2.2 Evaluation of political actors in COVID-19 measures: Mean comparison of ruling party supporters and others

	Ruling party supporters	*Others*	*t values*
Prime minister	3.58	2.59	16.02**
Central government	3.55	2.59	16.26**
Ruling party	3.49	2.51	17.21**
Opposition party	2.34	2.46	−2.25*
Expert subcommittee	4.03	3.61	6.85**
Prefectures	3.84	3.47	6.38**
Municipalities	3.78	3.39	6.64**
WHO	2.78	2.79	−0.25
N	595	1406	

* $p < .05$, ** $p < .01$.

score for non-supporters of the ruling party was around 2.5, indicating that they were more negative in their evaluation.

However, the opposition parties were even less appreciative. The mean rating was 2.34 among supporters of the ruling party, and 2.46 among the rest of the respondents, including supporters of the opposition, who also gave negative ratings. The continued dominance of the ruling party indicates that the opposition party did not have a strong presence in the COVID-19 measures.

Contrastingly, the expert subcommittee (Subcommittee on Novel Coronavirus Disease Control), comprised of medical experts, received a relatively high rating, averaging 4.03 for supporters of ruling parties and 3.61 for others.

Prefectures and municipalities likewise had higher mean values than central government actors, with a mean of 3.8 for supporters of the ruling party and 3.4 for all others. In terms of conflicts between the central and local governments, local governments were rated higher by citizens.[5] For instance, Hokkaido, Osaka, and Tokyo, which distinguished themselves in their COVID 19 measures, received scores of 4.1, 3.9, and 3.6, respectively, which were slightly higher than citizens' overall ratings.

The World Health Organization (WHO), an international organization, did not receive a very high rating, averaging 2.8.

Finally, Figure 2.2 displays the ratings of the policy formation process for both central and local governments to compare their differences. Across all items, the local government's mean score was approximately 3.0, while the central government's mean score was approximately 2.5, suggesting that the local government's evaluation was higher than that of the central government. In particular, the disparity was most significant for leadership, with a mean score of 3.4 for the local government and 2.6 for the central government. Individually, Hokkaido, Osaka, and Tokyo had relatively high mean scores of 4.3, 4.2, and 3.6, respectively, indicating that the local government evaluated the governor's performance highly.

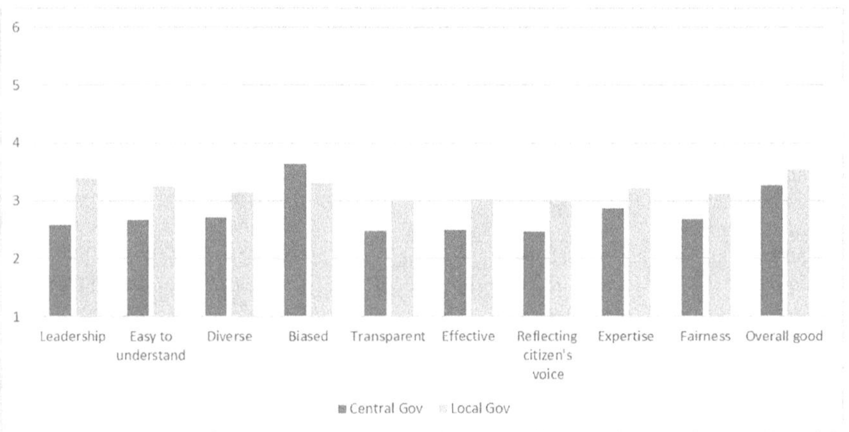

Figure 2.2 Evaluation of central and local government policy formation processes.

Conclusion

This chapter provides a comprehensive overview of the Japanese measures to combat the COVID-19 pandemic. During the Abe Administration, Japan faced the pandemic with the prime minister leading the policy formation. Due to the insufficient medical and digital capacity, proactive inspections were not conducted initially. Instead, the focus was on early detection and response to clusters.

Moreover, Japan did not enforce legally binding regulations on citizen behavior, relying instead on voluntary compliance. Despite the lack of coercion, Japanese citizens cooperated well. These points are essential to consider when making international comparisons.

However, the central government's policy was not always effective, as practical authority rested with the prefectures. The prefectural governors who opposed the central government's policy demonstrated remarkable performance. According to survey results, these governors were well-received by citizens, which may have provided a glimpse into the transformation of the power structure in Japan. The post-COVID-19 power structure, particularly the central-local relationship, remains an issue that requires attention in Japan.

Acknowledgment

The research in this chapter was supported by the Japan Society for the Promotion of Science (JSPS) Grants-in-Aid for Scientific Research [grant number 20H00061] and Murata Scientific Foundation.

Notes

1 The descriptions in this section are based on the author's reconstruction of the history of COVID-19 measures based on multiple sources. In particular, the author refers to the descriptions in the Asia Pacific Initiative (2020), Takenaka (2021), Kamata (2021), and the Yomiuri Shimbun Tokyo Research and Study Division (2022). The discussion is also similar to a previously published paper by the authors Yamamoto and Fujita (2023).
2 The meeting was subsequently abolished in July 2020, and a successor organization, "*Shingata Korona Uirusu Kansensho Taisaku Bunka Kai* (Subcommittee on Novel Coronavirus Disease Control)," was launched.
3 Novel Coronavirus Expert Meeting, "*Shingata Korona Uirusu Kansensho Taisaku no Kihon Hoshin no Gutaika ni Muketa Kenkai* [Opinion on the concretization of the basic policy for countermeasures against new coronavirus infection]," February 24, 2020, www.mhlw.go.jp/stf/seisakunitsuite/newpage_00006.html (Last viewed June 30, 2024)
4 In the survey that serves as the foundation for this book, Japanese respondents were asked about their perceptions of the COVID-19 measure in relation to the 2021 Lower House elections. According to the results, approximately half of the respondents (54.3%) indicated that they either "considered" or "considered a little" the COVID-19 measure when casting their votes. While COVID-19 was certainly a significant issue for voters, it did not appear to be a determining factor in their party selection.
5 A panel survey asking people to evaluate national and local government leaders also showed that local politicians were more highly rated. However, as vaccines began to be supplied, the gap narrowed over time (Mckelwein and Shibuya, 2023).

References

Altiparmakis, Argyrios, Abel Bojar, Sylvain Brouard, Martial Foucault, Hanspeter Kriesi, and Richard Nadeau. 2021. Pandemic politics: Policy evaluations of government responses to COVID-19. *West European Politics* 44(5–6): 1159–1179.

Asia Pacific Initiative (ed.). 2020. *Shingata Korona Taiou Minkan Rinji Chosakai: Chosa Kensho Hokokusho* [*Research and Verification Report by Private Sector ad hoc Investigative Committee for New Corona*]. Tokyo: Discover twenty-one.

Hanibuchi, Tomoya, Naoto Yabe, and Tomoki Nakaya. 2021. Who is staying home and who is not? Demographic, socioeconomic, and geographic differences in time spent outside the home during the COVID-19 outbreak in Japan. *Preventive Medicine Reports* 21: 101306.

Hata, Masaki. 2024. Self-restraint behavior and partisanship during the COVID-19 pandemic: Evidence from a list experiment in Japan. *Social Science Japan Journal* 27(2): 221–229.

Iijima, Wataru. 2021. *Jishuku* as a Japanese way for anti-COVID-19: Some basic reflections. *Historical Social Research* 33: 284–301.

Ito-Morales, Kyoko. 2022. Individual rights vs common good?: A case study on Japanese self-restraint (jishuku) and COVID-19. *Asian Studies* 10(1): 69–95.

Jørgensen, Frederik, Alexander Bor, Marie Fly Lindholt, and Michael Bang Petersen. 2021. Public support for government responses against COVID-19: Assessing levels and predictors in eight Western democracies during 2020. *West European Politics* 44(5–6): 1129–1158.

Kamata, Tsukasa, 2021. Korona taisaku wa Shuken ka bunken ka: Kuni mo chiho mo shikosakugo tsuduku [Is Corona measure centralized or decentralized?: Both the national and local governments continue to trial and error]. *Jichi Soken* 518: 1–34.

Kanai, Toshiyuki. 2021. *Korona Taisaku Ka no Kuni to Jichitai: Saigai Gyosei no Meiso to Heisoku* [*National and Local Governments in the Corona Countermeasure Disaster: Lost and Stuck in Disaster Administration*]. Tokyo: Chikuma Shobo.

Kashima, Saori, and Junyi Zhang. 2021. Temporal trends in voluntary behavioural changes during the early stages of the COVID-19 outbreak in Japan, *Public Health*, 192: 37–44.

Machidori, Satoshi. 2012. *Shusho Seiji no Seido Bunseki: Gendai Nihon Seiji no Kenryoku Kiban Keisei* [*Institutional Analysis of Prime Ministerial Politics: The Formation of the Power Base of Contemporary Japanese Politics*]. Tokyo: Chikura Shobo.

Machidori, Satoshi. 2020. *Seiji Kaikaku Saiko: Henbo wo Togeta Kokka no Kiseki* [*Rethinking Political Reform: The Trajectory of a State in Transformation*]. Tokyo: Shincho-sha.

Matsubara, Yu. 2021. Shingata korona uirusu kansensho no ryuko ni tomonau "Jishuku keisatsu" ni tsuite no Iichi kosatsu ["Jishuku-keisatsu (self-restraint police)" under the COVID-19 pandemic in Japan: Focusing on transformation of discursive space]. *Saigai to Kyosei* [*Disaster and Coexistence*] 5(1): 13–27.

McElwain, Kenneth Mori, and Yuya Shibuya, 2024, Joho to shinrai [Information and trust]. In Susumu Cato, Ryuichi Tanaka, and Kenneth Mori McElwain (eds.) *Pandemic to Shakai Kagaku: Posuto Korona kara Miete Kuru Mono* [*Pandemics and Social Science: Insights from Post-Covid Japan*]. Tokyo: Keiso Shobo pp.25–43.

Moon, M. Jae, Kohei Suzuki, Tae In Park, and Kentaro Sakuwa. 2021. A comparative study of COVID-19 responses in South Korea and Japan: Political nexus triad and policy responses. *International Review of Administrative Sciences* 87(3): 651–671.

Muto, Kaori, Isamu Yamamoto, Miwako Nagasu, Mikihito Tanaka, and Koji Wada. 2020. Japanese citizens' behavioral changes and preparedness against COVID-19: An online survey during the early phase of the pandemic, *PLoS One*, https://doi.org/10.1371/journal.pone.0234292

Nakakita, Koji. 2022. Choki antei seiken ni natta noha nazeka [How did it come to be a long-term government?] In Asia-Pacific Initiative (ed.). *Kensho Abe Seiken*: *Hoshu to Riarizumu no Seiji* [*The Abe Administration*: *The Politics of Conservatism and Realis*m]. Tokyo: Bungei Shunju.

Okada, Isamu, Itaru Yanagi, and Yoshiaki Kubo. 2022. COVID-19 Taisaku ni oite iryo shinrai ga kodo henyo ni oyobosu koka [The effect of trust in medical experts and system on behavioral changes in COVID-19 measures. *Senkyo Kenkyu* [*Japanese Journal of Electoral Studies*] 37(2): 37–56.

Reed, Steven R. 2022. Japanese electoral systems since 1947. In Robert Pekkanen and Saadia M. Pekkanen (eds.), *The Oxford Handbook of Japanese Politics*. New York: Oxford University Press, pp. 41–55.

Sasaki, Takeshi. 1999. *Seiji Kaikaku 1800 Nichi no Shinjitsu* [*The Truth about 1,800 Days of Political Reform*]. Tokyo: Kodansha.

Shaw, Rajib, Yong-Kyun Kim, and Jinling Hua. 2020. Governance, technology and citizen behavior in pandemic: Lessons from COVID-19 in East Asia. *Progress in Disaster Science* 6: 100090.

Shiroyama, Hideaki. 2020. Japan's response to the COVID-19. In Paul Joyce, Fabienne Maron, and Purshottama Sivanarain Reddy (eds.), *Good Public Governance in a Global Pandemic*. Brussels: IIAS-IISA, pp. 195–204.

Sunahara, Yosuke. 2020. Kuni no "Seiji shudo," chiho no "Seiji shudo" [National "political leadership," local "political leadership"]. *Chuo Koron* 134(8): 42–43.

Takenaka, Harukata. 2017. Seiken kotai wa Nani wo kaeta noka [What has the change in the government changed?]. In Haukata Takenaka (ed.), *Futasu no Seiken Kotai: Seisaku ha Kawatta Noka* [*Two Government Changes: Have Policies Changed?*]. Tokyo: Keiso Shobo, pp. 1–21.

Takenaka, Harukata. 2019. Expansion of the prime minister's power in the Japanese parliamentary system. *Asian Survey* 59(5): 844–869.

Takenaka, Harukata. 2021. *Korona Kiki no Seiji: Abe Seiken VS Chiji* [*Politics of the Corona Crisis: Abe Administration vs. Governors*].Tokyo: Chuo Koron Shinsha.

Taniguchi, Naoko, Plamen Akaliski, and Joonha Park. 2022. Korona ka ni okeru hitobito no "Fuan" to seijiteki akuta hyoka no kozo: "Kiki niokeru Kachi Henyo (Values in Crisis)" Kokusai Hikaku Chosa Dai 1 ha no Kekka kara [People's anxiety and evaluation of political actors under the COVID19 pandemic: Results from the first wave of the international comparative survey]. *Senkyo Kenkyu* [*Japanese Journal of Electoral Studies*] 37(2): 22–36.

Vardavas Constantine, Satomi Odani, Katerina Nikitara, and Nicholas Becuwe. 2021. Public perspective on the governmental response, communication and trust in the governmental decisions in mitigating COVID-19 early in the pandemic across the G7 countries. *Preventive Medicine Reports* 21: 101252.

Yamada, Masahiro. 2016. Seijikan [Political view]. In Ken'ichi Ikeda (ed.), *Nihonjin no Kangae kata, Sekai no Hito no Kangae kata: Sekai Kachikan Chosa kara Mieru mono* [*The Japanese Way of Thinking, the World Way of Thinking: What We Can See from the World Values Survey*]. Tokyo: Keiso Shobo, pp. 227–272.

Yamamoto, Hidehiro, and Taisuke Fujita. 2023. State-society relations under the COVID-19 disaster in Japan. In Jozef Oleński, Jeffrey Sachs, Masayuki Susai, Yannis Tsekouras, and Arjan Gjonça (eds.), *Handbook of Research on Socio-Economic Sustainability in the Post-Pandemic Era*, IGI Global [Hershey, PA], pp.139–157.

Yomiuri Shimbun Tokyo Research Division. 2022. *Hodo Kiroku Shingata Korona Uirusu Kansensho* [*The COVID-19 Timeline in Japan*].Tokyo: Yomiuri Shimbunsha.

3 The Paradox of Successful Government Responses to COVID-19 in South Korea

Youngho Cho and Gi-Woo Roh

Introduction

South Korea (hereafter, Korea) entered the COVID-19 pandemic on January 20, 2020. A month after the outbreak, the country's first death occurred, spiraling public fear about the pandemic. As in other countries, Korea's COVID-19 cases and deaths skyrocketed, focusing public attention on how the Korean government would respond to this terrifying crisis. The Korea Centers for Disease Control and Prevention (KCDC) immediately began holding daily press briefings in late January, and the Moon Jae-in administration elevated the COVID-19 risk level from "Alert" to the highest "Serious" and organized a government-wide response team in February.

Unlike other countries, which were not prepared and faced dire consequences from COVID-19, the Korean government quickly halted the massive transmission of the virus within two months. The number of COVID-19 cases dropped to single digits by late April. This approach, eventually termed "K-Quarantine," earned praise for its innovative measures such as drive-through testing, contact tracing, and QR code-based vaccine passes (Moon, 2020; Lim and Sohn, 2023). Notably, Korea did not enforce strict lockdowns but encouraged citizens' compliance by maintaining transparent communications and democratic procedures. In March 2022, daily cases of COVID-19 dramatically increased to more than 300,000 due to the Omicron variant. The situation started to improve in summer, however, because the variants were not as lethal and Korea's medical infrastructure was sufficient. The Korean government eased its preventive measures. In June 2023, the government lowered the COVID-19 risk level to "Alert" and lifted major quarantine guidelines. To date, the accumulative number of COVID-19 cases is about 38 million out of the 52 million population, with a fatality rate of 0.1%, which is the lowest in the world, demonstrating Korea's successful response to the pandemic crisis over the last 4 years.

The early success of K-Quarantine affected more than the sphere of public health, resulting in political spillovers. Korea held the 21st legislative elections on April 15, 2020, during the early period of the COVID-19 pandemic when public panic was escalating. In the fair and free elections, 66% of valid voters turned out

DOI: 10.4324/9781003495239-4

to cast their votes; the ruling Democratic Party and its allied parties won 180 seats, constituting 60% of the legislature. This landslide victory was unprecedented in legislative elections: No ruling party since the 1987 democratization had occupied three-fifths of the legislative seats. In addition, before the COVID-19 outbreak, the approval rating of President Moon Jae-in was below 50%, but during the pandemic it rose to over 70%. It seems that the initial success of the Moon Jae-in administration in combating COVID-19 boosted public confidence in the government. This increased political trust, in turn, further supported government efforts by securing Korean citizens' compliance (Moon et al., 2021).

However, the political success of the Moon Jae-in government did not last long. Within a year of the 2020 legislative elections, the ruling Democratic Party suffered a massive defeat in the by-elections of the Seoul and Pusan metropolitan mayors, triggering a lame-duck period for the Moon Jae-in government. Although President Moon Jae-in maintained an approval rating of about 40% even at the end of his term, the ruling Democratic Party failed to retain government power in the next presidential election, which was on March 9, 2022. Yoon Suk Yeol, who was once the prosecutor general appointed by Moon Jae-in but later disputed and challenged him, moved to the opposition People Power Party; he was nominated as their presidential candidate and was ultimately elected president.

Why did the Moon Jae-in government, despite its successful responses to the pandemic, face a lame-duck period, and why did his party fail to retain political power in the next elections? The Moon Jae-in government was unusual in two respects. Since the 1987 democratization, Korean governments have typically changed every ten years between conservative and progressive parties, but the progressive Moon government handed power to the opposition party in just five years. Furthermore, the Moon Jae-in government emerged from the massive 2016–2017 candlelight protests that ended the Park Geun-hye conservative government. Korean citizens had high expectations for the Moon Jae-in government, and early approval ratings exceeded 80%. The successful response to COVID-19 seemed to uphold the legitimacy of Moon Jae-in. Despite these positive factors, however, his government crumbled in early 2021 and failed to secure political power.

This chapter aims to elucidate how the Moon Jae-in government responded to the COVID-19 pandemic so successfully and why the positive response to these policies did not translate into long-term political success. In exploring this, we focus on government trust during the pandemic period. Political trust is crucial in times of crisis because citizens with high levels of such trust are more likely to voluntarily comply with governmental policies aiming to manage the crisis, thereby influencing policy success. Furthermore, government trust is a key component of state-society relations because it facilitates collaboration between civil society and government when dealing with crises. As Putnam (1993) aptly pointed out, individuals who are confident in their government allow it more flexibility in implementing challenging measures and are more likely to tolerate the inconvenience associated with those measures.

Because government trust is dynamic rather than static, we trace its changes during the COVID-19 crisis in Korea. Changes in government trust reflected how the Moon Jae-in government performed during the pandemic period. To examine these changes, we used a panel survey: The first and second waves were conducted in July 2020 and February 2021, respectively. Previous studies that relied on one-time surveys or cross-national surveys were limited in exploring the dynamic nature of government trust. By using a panel survey to examine changes in government trust, we aim to shed light on Korea's response to the COVID-19 crisis and its impact on Korean politics. Our findings will have substantial implications for understanding the changing yet enduring nature of state-society relations in Korea.

This chapter is organized as follows. The next section critically reviews political trust and the pandemic crisis. The third section discusses the theoretical perspectives of rational citizens and multi-dimensional performance evaluations, emphasizing how these factors interact to influence government trust and its changes. The fourth section presents empirical results and provides interpretations. The final section summarizes the major findings and draws implications for state-society relations in Korea.

Literature Review: Government Trust and the Pandemic Crisis

Government trust is relevant in both policy implementation and democratic politics (Citrin and Stoker, 2018; Putnam, 1993). Public trust in government is generally conceived as a resource for authorities to plan and implement policies. For government policies to succeed, authorities must minimize civic resistance and ensure citizens' compliance. Theoretically, government trust reduces transaction costs, which inevitably arise in the process of policy-making and implementation. As Hetherington (1998) pointed out, high political trust creates a policy environment in which leaders are likely to succeed. Conversely, low trust tends to limit both the scope of leaders' actions and their flexibility in decision-making.

Beyond the policy domain, government trust plays a role in political dynamics in a representative democracy (Chanley et al., 2000; Pharr and Putnam, 2000). Although changes in political trust do not necessarily lead to government turnover in authoritarian regimes, political trust is a crucial factor in holding government accountable to voters and ensuring it is responsive to public demands in a modern democracy (Putnam, 1993). It is because political trust is dynamic by nature, and this change is often a precursor to government turnover, making it difficult for leaders to ignore public concerns and demands. Therefore, political trust is an integral component of state-society relations.

The relevance of government trust becomes particularly prominent during various types of crises (Chanley, 2002). In the context of a pandemic, crises occur unexpectedly, and both citizens and government are often ill-prepared. As damage and fear spread, public attention focuses on government actions and measures because the modern state is designed and expected to protect citizens' lives and property. Moreover, as ordinary citizens cannot effectively respond to pandemic diseases or manage the economic and social crises caused by a pandemic, their concerns about and expectations for government actions increase. These heightened expectations and the urgency of crisis management make government responses to the pandemic crises particularly salient. As a result, government performance is likely to be the most significant determinant of political trust, whereas other factors such as socio-economic backgrounds and partisanship tend to have diminished impact.

These theoretical expectations are reflected in the literature on political trust during the COVID-19 crisis. The public's fear spiraled and persisted until various COVID-19 vaccines were approved and large-scale vaccination campaigns began in late 2020 and early 2021. During the first year of the COVID-19 outbreak, the rally-round-the-flag-effect on government trust was observed across countries (Bækgaard et al., 2020; Kallemose et al., 2023; Schraff, 2021; Van der Meer et al., 2023). For example, Bol and his colleagues (2020) found evidence of increased trust in government in Europe during the COVID-19 pandemic. Similar trends were reported in China (Su et al., 2021), Canada (Bourgeois et al., 2020), Spain (Belchior and Teixeira, 2023), and the Middle East (Beschel, 2021). Korea also followed this trend (Roh et al., 2021).

However, rising government trust was not universal; it varied across countries and groups. In particular, Suhay and colleagues (2022) traced public trust in federal, state, and local governments in the United States from March to October 2020 and found a downward trend. Negative perceptions of pandemic management, particularly in the United States, led to a decline in political trust among US citizens (Aassve et al., 2024). Using cross-national surveys of 57 countries, Rieger and Wang (2022) found that effective government responses were associated with high political trust.

Furthermore, government trust varied among different groups. The most significant gap appeared across partisan lines, which is understandable, given that President Trump downplayed the severity of COVID-19, did not implement timely preventive measures at the federal level, and placed much of the burden for responding to the pandemic onto states and localities while blaming China (James et al., 2022). This demonstrates that responses to COVID-19 became politicized in the United States, despite increasingly clear findings from scientific and public health communities.

Overall, these empirical studies expand our current understanding of political trust and the COVID-19 crisis and support existing findings about the nexus between natural disasters and politics (Carlin et al., 2014; Healy and Malhotra, 2009). For example, the positive changes in political trust make sense because various governments quickly took preventive campaigns, despite differences in their approaches and levels of quarantine, which aligns with the performance theory of political trust (Miller, 1974; Van der Meer and Hakhverdian, 2017). In this context, the politicization and polarization in the US response to the pandemic was largely due to President Trump, eventually leading to a decline in government trust (Suhay et al., 2022).

In addition, individual fear of contracting COVID-19 was likely to be higher among senior citizens than among younger people, and the former shows higher levels of political support for the government than the latter (Van der Meer et al., 2023). The divergence in government trust between younger and older generations was also found in Britain (Parsons and Wiggins, 2020).

Although prior studies highlight the importance and dynamic of government trust with regard to the COVID-19 pandemic, they have some limitations. Trust in government increased in the early period of the pandemic, easing government burdens, but it started to decline across countries. Existing research has not focused enough on this changing nature of political trust, which is partially due to limitations in survey data. With a few notable exceptions (Aassve et al., 2024; Suhay et al., 2022; Van der Meer et al., 2023), most studies employ one-shot national surveys or cross-national surveys (Bækgaard et al., 2020; Bol et al., 2020; Ji et al., 2024; Kallemose et al., 2023; Rieger and Wang, 2022). When comparing government trust before and during the pandemic, these studies confirmed that political trust increased in response to the implementation of a government's preventive campaigns. However, they do not explain why political trust did not persist during the pandemic and began to decline. More importantly, they are limited in accounting for the dynamics of political trust whereby individual citizens evaluate various aspects of government performance at different time points with varying levels of issue salience during the COVID-19 crisis. Individual citizens focus on different dimensions of government performance depending on their concerns and expectations, and this evaluation is a key mechanism of political trust.

This study aims to elucidate how political trust changed in response to the Korean government's handling of the COVID-19 crisis and other significant issues. Although the COVID-19 crisis was the most critical and urgent issue in 2020, it was not the only issue that the government had to address. In addition, the conditions surrounding COVID-19 varied over time due to factors such as vaccination progress and changing rates of daily cases and deaths. Therefore, we utilized a panel survey to examine Korea's experience with the pandemic.

Theoretical Discussion: Rational Voters and Multidimensional Performance Evaluation

This research is premised on the notion that ordinary voters are rational and politics is far distant from the everyday lives of rational voters (Popkin, 1991). The perceived distance between voters and politics tends to increase as a country grows in geographical size and population. Because modern democracy relies on representative government and popular elections, most voters focus on private life with the protection of civil rights between elections. Voters' attention and participation generally increase during election periods, as elections are a primary means by which parties and candidates mobilize and voters give consent to their elected representatives. Even during elections, however, individual voters have limited knowledge and sophistication.

As John Zaller (1992) pointed out, ordinary voters do not possess sufficient resources to pay close attention to politics. Nonetheless, it does not mean that they do not evaluate and judge government activities (Bartels, 1996). Because rational voters tend to be cognitive misers using their limited time and resources efficiently, they assess government performance by considering different levels of salience across various issues. Every government faces a variety of issues that require attention, and their relative importance can vary depending on the situation and environment (Miller, 1974; Chanley, 2002; Hetherington and Rudolph, 2015). Typically, the most salient problem discussed in the mass media and public discourse becomes the standard by which citizens assess governments. Economic performance is generally a key factor in retrospective voting (Healy and Malhotra, 2013), whereas foreign policy and security become central when a country faces threats or attacks. For example, Chanley (2002) showed that the rally-round-the-flag effect emerged right after the 9/11 terrorist attacks on the United States in 2001, leading to a surge in public attention and trust in the government in response to the Bush administration's war on terror. At that time, foreign policy and security overshadowed other issues.

The idea that voters are rational and cognitive misers indicates they evaluate government performance in a multidimensional manner. The outbreak of the COVID-19 pandemic suddenly caused public fear, directing all citizens' focus toward the government's response because they could not address the pandemic individually. However, once the threat and fear moderated, ordinary voters naturally considered government performance in terms of other issues. This is an example of why government trust changes and democratic politics remains accountable: The government cannot consistently achieve the best results across all issues, and opposition parties tend to focus on those issue areas in which the government underperforms or makes mistakes. As Dahl (1971) noted, "a key characteristic of a democracy is the continuing responsiveness of the government to the preferences of its citizens" (p. 1), therefore, democracy is never static but dynamic as democratic governments continually face new and puzzling issues.

We expect that three major issues push to the forefront for Korean citizens and influence their evaluation of government performance: COVID-19 pandemic, the economy, and real estate. First, the government response to the pandemic is considered primarily salient. When the Korean government relaxed major preventive measures in June 2023, the pandemic had been a persistent issue for both the government and the Korean people since its outbreak. However, public concern about the pandemic was likely influenced by the initial government response, as the widespread transmission depended on how quickly the government could ramp up social and medical preparedness to contain it. Otherwise, the pandemic could spiral out of control, trapping both the government and citizens in a vicious circle of underperformance and declining trust. Therefore, we believe that Korean people would adjust political trust according to their evaluation of the government's early response.

Second, the economy is a key issue because it affects the everyday lives of Korean citizens, much as it does in other countries. As Korea transitions into an advanced industrial economy, its growth rate has slowed, regardless of which party is in power. National economic conditions have been a consistent concern for ordinary Koreans, and the salience of these conditions increased because the pandemic negatively affected middle- and lower-class Koreans in terms of income, reductions in working hours, and unemployment. Nonetheless, between 2019 and 2021 Korea's economic growth was 3.1%, which was twice the average of the OECD countries (OECD, 2023). More significantly, in June 2020, the OECD projected Korea to be the least-affected economy, which alleviated severe economic concerns among Korean people and boosted their national pride. As a result, we anticipate that, aware of these international and domestic assessments, Korean citizens would revise their confidence in the government.

Finally, we consider that real estate was a critical issue for Korean citizens, regardless of whether or not they owned a house. Rising housing prices were burdensome for homeowners due to property tax increases, and the Moon Jae-in government announced additional tax hikes proportional to real estate prices. This policy, the normalization of property tax, irritated wealthy Koreans whose income changed little during the pandemic. Skyrocketing real estate prices also meant that those without a house were likely to lose an opportunity to purchase one, leading to a sense of relative deprivation. Throughout the Moon Jae-in administration (2017–2022), real estate prices continued to rise despite the government's repeated promises to intervene and control speculators. Real estate prices moved in the opposite direction of government announcements and interventions. Notably, the average price for Seoul apartments doubled from 600 million to 1,200 million KRW during his term (Kwon, 2021). The price of a Seoul apartment is of particular significance in Korea because 52% of the population lives in Seoul and the capital area, and many desire to own an apartment in Seoul. In addition, soaring real estate prices were a crucial issue because 64% of nonfinancial assets in 2021 were household wealth (Korea Financial Investment Association, 2022). This is significant when compared with other countries: The proportion is 29% in the US, 37% in Japan, and 46% in the UK. Real estate comprises 75% of the nonfinancial wealth among Korean households. Therefore, we posit that the performance evaluation of real estate negatively affected government trust among Korean citizens.

We believe that performance evaluation is a key factor in political trust among Korean citizens. As Choi and Woo (2016) and Wang (2016) found, East Asian people prioritize tangible results over other factors, such as procedural justice, when judging politics and governments. Therefore, we conceive the pandemic, the economy, and real estate to be the most salient issues. These are not the only significant issues that the Korean government addresses. For example, security and North Korea have been persistent concerns in Korea. However, North Korean aggression was not particularly provocative during 2020–2021 because North Korea implemented strict lockdowns within its territory as well as along the border. We do not include other issues because we believe that these three are sufficient to illustrate how Koreans evaluate government performance and how their political trust changes.

Furthermore, we argue that salient issues can shift the perception of Korean people. Citizens tend to focus on the most salient issue and expect the government to direct its resources accordingly. However, when the most pressing issue, in this case COVID-19, becomes less severe, it gives way to newly emerging or enduring issues such as the economy and real estate. It is natural for Korean citizens to follow these issues and adjust their political trust based on how the government addresses them. This is why government trust changes and why politics is dynamic and accountable in Korea's democracy. We apply this theoretical framework to shed new light on government trust and political dynamics during the first year of COVID-19.

Analytical Results: The Paradox of Government Success against COVID-19 in Korea

How did Korea respond to COVID-19 in such a quick and successful manner? Does this success contribute to government trust among Korean citizens? When Korean people adjusted their confidence in the government during the pandemic, what other factors influenced the change? To answer these questions, we conducted an online panel survey via the internet and cellphone. The first wave asked 2,545 Korean citizens about their perceptions of COVID-19, their reactions to government responses, and their political attitudes from June 24 to July 1, 2020. July 2020 was a period when Korea had successfully contained the massive transmission of coronavirus and established a robust statewide response against the pandemic, yet public fear did not subside because vaccine development was uncertain.

The second wave surveyed 1,832 respondents from March 17 to March 23, 2021. Although 713 respondents dropped out after the first wave, about 72% of the original respondents participated in the second panel survey. Considering that most Korean mass surveys typically have about 1,000 respondents, this panel survey had nearly twice as many respondents as other social surveys. As a nationwide survey, proportional quotas were allocated by gender and generations within 17 administrative regions on the basis of the Korean population census. Therefore, the panel survey data are reliable and valid for ascertaining government trust and its changes during the COVID-19 period.

Before examining the empirical results, it is important to explain how Korea coped with the COVID-19 crisis and how the approval ratings for President Moon Jae-in changed. Because the lame-duck period for the Moon Jae-in government began with the loss in the April 2021 by-elections for the Seoul and Pusan metropolitan mayors, the first year of COVID 19 was crucial in determining the final year of the presidential term and the government turnover in the 2022 presidential election. Before the April 2021 by-elections, conservative parties in Korea were fragile and fragmented because the large 2016–2017 candlelight protest that resulted in the impeachment of former president Park Geun-hye led to their collapse. Although the conservative parties united to form the People Power Party for the April 2020 legislative elections, the United Conservative Party experienced a historic loss, winning less than 40% of the seats. However, the People Power Party began to recover with its victory in the by-elections for the Seoul and Pusan metropolitan mayors in April 2021, ultimately leading to government turnover in the March 2022 presidential election. Given these events, it is puzzling that the Moon Jae-in government, which began with unusually high popularity and displayed a successful response to COVID-19, failed to achieve political success after 2020.

Figure 3.1 shows weekly cases of COVID-19 and the approval ratings of President Moon Jae-in from February 2020 to March 2021. It appears that weekly cases

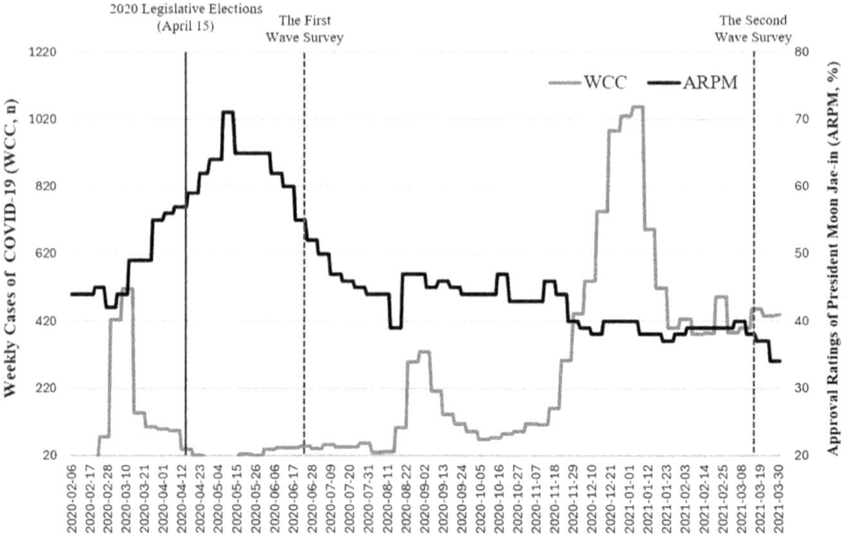

Figure 3.1 Weekly cases of COVID-19 and approval ratings of President Moon Jae-in, February 2020–March 2021.

Source: WHO COVID-19 Dashboard (processed by Our World in Data); Gallup Korea Daily Opinion.

and approval ratings tend to move in opposite directions, respectively. According to Figure 3.1, the approval ratings of President Moon Jae-in were slightly above 40% in February 2020 and started to increase in March. Although the figure does not indicate, the approval ratings of Moon Jae-in remained steady at around 45% throughout 2019. The confirmed cases of COVID-19 soared in late February 2020 when a growing number of new cases were traced to illegal gatherings and events at the Shincheonji Church of Jesus, which mainstream churches considered a cult. Infection cases continued to rise until the first week of March but were significantly controlled through the late summer: The cases dropped to about ten in late April and early May.

How did Korea respond to the pandemic? The Moon Jae-in government began daily press briefings as early as January 2020 and pushed transparent communications, sharing the changing situations and preventive guidelines via mass media. The government opted against forceful lockdowns, instead persuading citizens to comply and expanding the government-wide response system to include medical and societal levels. At the same time, the Korean government implemented preventive guidelines such as travel restrictions, quarantine, contact tracing, and social distancing, which quickly took hold. The Korean government also distributed disaster relief funds and maintained medical and social infrastructure to combat the pandemic. These efforts would not have been successful without citizens' compliance, and Korea's response (often referred to as K-Quarantine) earned worldwide praise. Finally, as Figure 3.1 illustrates, the number of cases fell to single digits in late April. Although cases and deaths fluctuated, the social and medical infrastructures were sufficiently developed to control the subsequent impacts of the pandemic.

Korea's success story was widely circulated in mass media, resulting in political spillovers. The approval rating for President Moon Jae-in rose to 57% in the third week of April 2020 when the ruling Democratic Party won a landslide victory, securing 180 out of the 300 legislative seats. In early May, Moon Jae-in's job approval peaked at 71%, whereas only 21% disapproved and 10% remained neutral.

How did the Korean government upgrade these various measures so quickly? The answer lies in the medical and political lessons from the past failure of the Korean government's response to Middle East Respiratory Syndrome (MERS) in 2015 (Kang et al., 2020; J.-H. Kim et al., 2020; Moon, 2020; Park and Chung, 2021). The MERS outbreak occurred in Korea in late May 2015 and spread in early summer. The Park Geun-hye government failed to respond actively to the MERS pandemic, initially withholding information about the disease from the public. Instead, the police warned that those leaking information about MERS or sharing it online while raising doubts and concerns about the lack of government response would be investigated and punished (Cho, 2019). This caused public fear and anxiety, especially among mothers with young children and babies. The Korean government initiated a belated administrative and medical response 2 months after the outbreak, leading to 38 deaths out of the 184 affected individuals, making Korea the most affected country after Saudi Arabia.

This outcome was shocking at the time because pandemic diseases such as smallpox, measles, and typhoid fever had virtually disappeared in the 1970s, and no new pandemic had emerged in Korea before the MERS outbreak in 2015. Korea's late, rigid, narrow, and passive response to MERS had political consequences, with Park Geun-hye's approval ratings plummeting from 40% to 29% within a month after the outbreak. This collective experience contributed to the ruling party's loss in the 2016 legislative elections (Chung, 2016).

The lessons from MERS are both medical and political, given the human and political damages. First, both MERS and COVID-19 are human coronaviruses, causing respiratory symptoms and damage; COVID-19 is short for *coronavirus disease 2019*. Thus, preventive guidelines and various responses during COVID-19 were similar to those implemented at medical, governmental, and societal levels during the 2015 MERS outbreak: People in Korea started using hand sanitizer and wearing masks, and Korea's government re-introduced contact tracing and quarantine first used during MERS (Kang et al., 2020; J.-H. Kim et al., 2020).

In addition, those high-ranking officials at the Center for Disease Control who were responsible for the MERS failure faced disciplinary punishments. Of these, two officials, Jeong Eun-Kyeong and Kwon Jun Wook, played a leading role in the government response to COVID-19, spearheading preventive measures. Jeong Eun-Kyeong became the first Commissioner of the Korea Disease Control and Prevention Agency (KDCA) in 2020, which was expanded and upgraded from the

Korea Center for Disease Control (KCDC). Moreover, Korea maintained medical preparedness and preventive measures against MERS until October 22, 2018, and kept the alarm system to detect and respond to MERS. Therefore, decisions during the COVID-19 pandemic could be seen as an extension of the MERS experience in Korea.

Second, the MERS outbreak provided political lessons (Cho, 2019). It was not the first failure in government disaster management under President Park Geun-hye's leadership. The ferry MV Sewol sank on the morning of April 16, 2014, a route from Incheon to Jeju. Of 476 passengers and crew, 304 died in the disaster, including around 250 high school students on a graduation trip to Jeju. The Park Geun-hye government did not actively respond to this disaster but minimized its responsibility, eventually drawing public outrage and criticism. Learning from the fact that these two failures contributed to the decline of the Park Geun-hye government, the Moon Jae-in government pursued active responses to natural disasters and the COVID-19 pandemic. For example, President Moon Jae-in ordered government-wide responses to the 2017 Pohang earthquake and the large 2018 forest fires in Gangneung-Donghae on the East Coast. Moon Jae-in's approach to COVID-19 was statewide, whereas Park Geun-hye's response to MERS remained at the ministry level. The Moon Jae-in government response was active and transparent, whereas the Park Geun-hye government response was passive and somewhat authoritarian: The former relied on public persuasion, whereas the latter used coercive warnings and threats.

Did Korea's successful response to COVID-19 lead to political returns in terms of government trust? The survey asked respondents how much they trusted the government with four responses ranging from "Do not trust at all" to "Trust well." For simplicity, we dichotomized those four responses into two categories: trust and distrust.

As presented in Figure 3.2, those who trusted the government were as high as 60% in the first wave, but this declined to 46% in the second wave. Correspondingly, those who distrusted the government increased by 14%. This is a significant result, but it hides the micro-variation of government trust changes at the individual level. Indeed, about 23% of the respondents changed their government trust. Among them, 4% of the respondents shifted from distrusting the government to trusting it, while 19% changed from trusting the government to distrusting it. This suggests that government trust is dynamic, and a panel survey is necessary to trace these changes.

Why did citizens' trust in the government change so significantly in a negative way? We argue that different issues have varying levels of salience at different points in time (Miller, 1974; Van der Meer and Hakhverdian, 2017). Although COVID-19 remained a critical issue, other concerns such as the economy and real estate became more prominent in the eyes of the Korean people. Changes in government trust likely reflected the government's performance across these three issue areas in a balanced manner. Therefore, we first examine how Korean citizens assess government performance in response to these issues and then explore the link between performance evaluation and changes in government trust. Unfortunately,

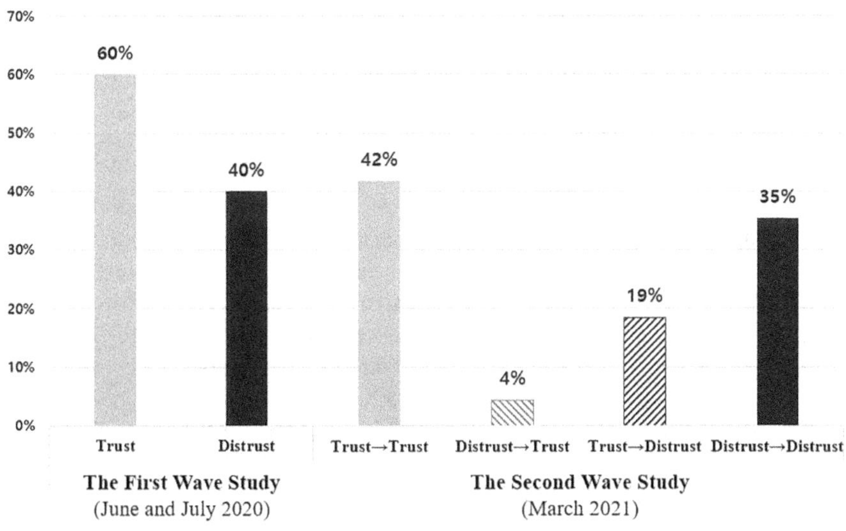

Figure 3.2 Government trust and change between the first and second waves of the panel survey.

Table 3.1 Korean public evaluation on government performance to COVID-19, the economy, and real estate

	Positive (%)	*Neutral (%)*	*Negative (%)*
COVID-19	70	14	16
The economy	34	20	46
Real estate	17	13	70

the first wave did not include questions regarding the government's response to the economy and real estate but these were included in the second wave. Thus, we will focus our examination on the change in government trust between these two waves. This approach is valid to answer why the Moon Jae-in government's successful response to COVID-19 failed to achieve political success after 2020 because government trust neither changed nor rebounded significantly after the second wave.

Table 3.1 shows how Korean people evaluated their government's response to COVID-19, the economy, and real estate during the second wave. The key finding is that the performance evaluation differs greatly between COVID-19 and real estate. For example, 70% of the respondents were negative about the government's response to real estate, whereas the same proportion was positive about its response to COVID-19. Considering that respondents had the option to answer a neutral response, seven out of ten expressed a negative view on the issue of real estate. This negative evaluation was understandable because the price of Seoul apartments nearly doubled in 2021 and housing prices rose in other regions, despite the government's continuing promises to control real estate prices. Those who believed in the government's promises and waited to buy a new apartment or house felt betrayed, whereas those who owned apartments faced proportionally increased property tax. Finally, public evaluation of the government's response to economy was mixed: 46% had a negative view and 34% had a positive view.

It seems that changes in government trust after the first wave were likely to reflect public evaluation of these three issues. When Figure 3.2 and Table 3.1 are considered together, it suggests that positive evaluations of the government's COVID-19 response supported government trust, whereas negative evaluations contributed to its decline. Did performance evaluations on these three issues predict government trust changes? Figure 3.3 shows the relationship between performance evaluation and government trust change. The net change between the first and second waves was -14%. Table 3.1 indicates the distribution of negative changes across the three issues.

According to Figure 3.3, a positive evaluation of government's performance on COVID-19 offset the negative evaluation in terms of trust change. On the other hand, negative evaluations of the economy and real estate had a greater impact on trust change, overwhelming any positive effects. In particular, the decline in government trust was above the average -14% in three groups: those who were neutral or negative on economy and those negative on real estate. Given that those who negatively evaluated the government's performance on COVID-19, the economy, and the real estate were 16%, 46%, and 70%, respectively, it is reasonable to conclude

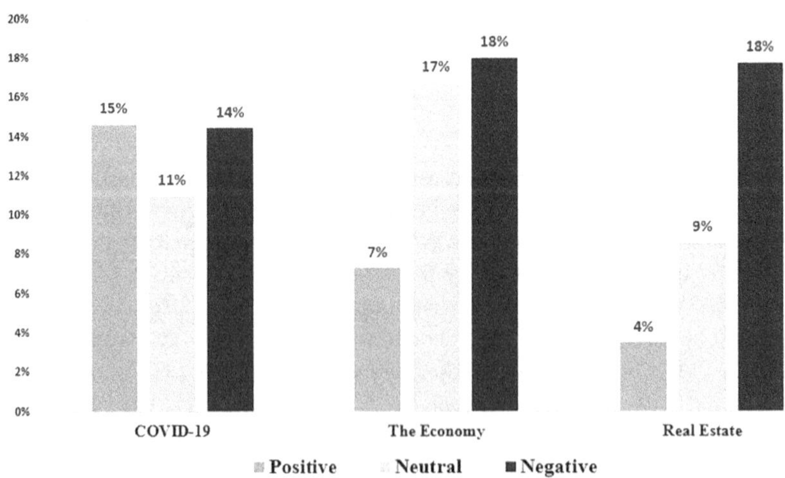

Figure 3.3 Relationships between performance evaluation and government trust change (net change: −14%).

that the detrimental effects on trust change were in the opposite order: real estate, economy, and COVID-19.

These findings support the initial expectation that the government's response to real estate led to a decrease in political trust, whereas its successful response to COVID-19 maintained it. Our survey did not ask respondents for reasons behind their trust and distrust, so we attempt to ascertain statistical correlations between performance evaluation and changes in political trust. However, the *Gallup* weekly survey asked for reasons behind the approval and disapproval ratings for President Moon Jae-in during the two periods in which the first and second waves of the panel survey were conducted (Gallup Korea, 2020, 2021). The *Gallup* survey indicates that the most frequent reasons for approval and disapproval ratings were COVID-19 (33%) and North Korea (19%) during the former period and COVID-19 (22%) and real estate (37%) during the latter period. These results support our argument that these three issues have different levels of salience at different times, and Korean citizens used these to evaluate government performance and adjust their political trust accordingly.

Descriptive statistics from Figures 3.1–3.3 and Table 3.1 provide insights into how the Moon Jae-in government responded to COVID-19, demonstrating that this successful response led to government trust. They also offer reasons why government trust declined at the aggregate level. However, descriptive statistics alone do not provide robust evidence for two reasons. The first is that evidence at the aggregate level does not necessarily align with valid inference at the individual level, which is associated with an ecological fallacy. The second is the problem of model specification with omitted variables. The descriptive statistics presented in this chapter show direct relations between performance evaluation and government trust change but they do not control other predictors known in the existing literature. This problem might cause either an optical illusion regarding the relations or inflated effects of specific variables.

To avoid the possibility of ecological fallacy and to address the problem of omitted variables, we conducted a multivariate regression with three independent variables: performance evaluations for COVID-19, the economy, and real estate. We also included control variables, classified into three categories: political, socioeconomic, and demographic. The political control variables are ideology and party identifications (People Power Party, minor parties, and those not affiliated—the baseline group is the ruling Democratic Party). The socioeconomic variables are life satisfaction, interpersonal trust, educational attainment, subjective class identification, and objective class position combining both monthly income and assets. The final demographic variables are direct damage from COVID-19, psychological stress from COVID-19, female dummy, generations, and residence (Kyungsang and Jeolla).

Because we are interested in the decline of government trust but only include the two questions about performance evaluation on the economy and real estate in the second wave, we take two sequential steps. First, we regress the government trust score from the second wave on independent and control variables while including the government trust score from the first wave. This approach indirectly controls the persistent effect of government trust between the two waves, allowing us to examine what factors sustain or lower government trust in the second wave. Since government trust ranges from 1 to 4, we use ordinal logistic regression. Second, we subtract the government trust score of the first wave from that of the second wave to create a variable of government trust change. Although this variable mathematically ranges from −3 to 3, its actual distribution is skewed toward negative numbers: The mean value is −0.24. We employ linear regression of government trust change on independent and control variables, excluding government trust from the first wave. This step helps determine whether the decline in government trust occurred at the individual level, at the aggregate level, or at both levels between the two waves.

Table 3.2 reports analytical results on government trust and its change as shown in the second wave. There are several notable findings. First of all, the four models of Step 1 show that all three variables of performance evaluation of COVID-19, the economy, and real estate are statically significant in determining government trust, with substantial effects. Those who positively evaluated COVID-19, the economy, and real estate are likely to have confidence in the government. On the contrary, those who negatively assessed performance are likely to show distrust. Given that performance evaluations for these three issues are broadly positive, moderate, and negative in that order, it is reasonable to conclude that a positive evaluation of COVID-19 contributed to sustained government trust, whereas a negative evaluation of real estate led to distrust in the government.

Second, among the political variables, party identifications stand out given that both those unaffiliated and those supporting the opposition parties are likely to show lower government trust compared with supporters of the ruling Democratic Party. A substantial gap in government trust is observed between those unaffiliated and supporters of the ruling party, indicating that the former group turned away from the government in the second wave. Other control variables are either statistically insignificant or have a small effect.

Third, the empirical results reported in the four models of Step 2 also support our theoretical expectations. The performance evaluation of COVID-19 is not statistically associated with changes in government trust. Given that this variable positively correlates with government trust in the second wave, it indicates that a positive evaluation of COVID-19 sustained government trust between the two waves. On the other hand, the performance evaluations on the economy and real estate are correlated with changes in government trust in Models 6 and 7. In the extended Model 8, the performance evaluation of the economy becomes statistically insignificant, but the performance evaluation of real estate remains a significant factor in the decline of government trust. Because negative evaluations of real estate dominated, it appears that this factor contributed directly to the decrease in government trust in the second wave.

Fourth, as expected, government trust waned among those unaffiliated compared to those supportive of the ruling Democratic Party. Furthermore, the value of the constant is −0.44, indicating that government trust substantially decreased after the first wave. Given that government trust has a three-point scale and their standard

Table 3.2 Analytical results of government trust and its change

VARIABLES	*Step 1. D.V.: Government Trust (Ordinal Logistic Regression)*				*Step 2. D.V.: Government Trust Change (Linear Regression)*			
	Model 1	*Model 2*	*Model 3*	*Model 4*	*Model 5*	*Model 6*	*Model 7*	*Model 8*
Government Trust (Wave 1)	1.86***	1.85***	1.97***	1.70***				
	(0.10)	(0.10)	(0.10)	(0.11)				
Performance Evaluation: COVID-19	**0.36*****			**0.23*****	**0.01**	**−0.02**	**−0.01**	**−0.01**
	(0.03)			**(0.04)**	**(0.01)**	**(0.01)**	**(0.01)**	**(0.01)**
Performance Evaluation: The Economy		**0.39*****		**0.18*****		**0.04*****		**0.01**
		(0.03)		**(0.04)**		**(0.01)**		**(0.01)**
Performance Evaluation: Real Estate			**0.34*****	**0.20*****			**0.04*****	**0.03*****
			(0.03)	**(0.03)**			**(0.01)**	**(0.01)**
Ideology	−0.085*	−0.08*	−0.09*	−0.06	0.01	0.01	0.01	0.01
	(0.036)	(0.04)	(0.04)	(0.04)	(0.01)	(0.01)	(0.01)	(0.01)
Ruling Democratic Party (Baseline)								
People Power Party	−1.30***	−1.07***	−1.21***	−0.94***	−0.13*	−0.07	−0.07	−0.06
	(0.24)	(0.23)	(0.23)	(0.24)	(0.07)	(0.07)	(0.07)	(0.07)
Minor parties	−0.84***	−0.59**	-0.65***	−0.55**	−0.06	−0.02	−0.01	−0.01
	(0.19)	(0.20)	(0.20)	(0.20)	(0.05)	(0.05)	(0.05)	(0.05)
Unaffiliated	−1.21***	−1.05***	−1.09***	−0.92***	−0.17***	−0.12**	−0.10**	−0.10*

(*Continued*)

Table 3.2 (Continued)

VARIABLES	*Step 1. D.V.: Government Trust (Ordinal Logistic Regression)*				*Step 2. D.V.: Government Trust Change (Linear Regression)*			
	Model 1	*Model 2*	*Model 3*	*Model 4*	*Model 5*	*Model 6*	*Model 7*	*Model 8*
	(0.15)	(0.16)	(0.16)	(0.16)	(0.04)	(0.04)	(0.04)	(0.04)
Life Satisfaction	0.02	0.01	0.03	−0.00	0.00	−0.00	0.00	−0.00
	(0.03)	(0.03)	(0.03)	(0.04)	(0.01)	(0.01)	(0.01)	(0.01)
Interpersonal Trust	0.36***	0.29**	0.18	0.23*	0.06*	0.05	0.04	0.04
	(0.10)	(0.09)	(0.09)	(0.10)	(0.03)	(0.03)	(0.03)	(0.03)
Education	−0.06	−0.03	−0.02	−0.01	−0.02	−0.01	−0.01	−0.01
	(0.06)	(0.06)	(0.06)	(0.06)	(0.02)	(0.02)	(0.02)	(0.02)
Subjective Class Identification	0.14	0.10	0.08	0.11	0.04	0.04	0.03	0.03
	(0.08)	(0.08)	(0.08)	(0.08)	(0.02)	(0.02)	(0.02)	(0.02)
Objective Class Position	−0.13**	−0.10*	−0.07	−0.08	−0.03*	−0.03*	−0.02	−0.02
	(0.04)	(0.04)	(0.04)	(0.04)	(0.01)	(0.01)	(0.01)	(0.01)
Damage from COVID-19	−0.10	−0.03	−0.07	−0.03	−0.01	−0.00	−0.01	−0.00
	(0.07)	(0.08)	(0.07)	(0.08)	(0.02)	(0.02)	(0.02)	(0.02)
Psychological Stress from COVID-19	−0.01	−0.01	−0.02	−0.03	0.01	0.01	0.00	0.00
	(0.05)	(0.05)	(0.05)	(0.06)	(0.02)	(0.02)	(0.02)	(0.02)
Female Dummy	−0.08	−0.15	−0.16	−0.14	−0.04	−0.05	−0.05	−0.05
	(0.10)	(0.11)	(0.11)	(0.11)	(0.03)	(0.03)	(0.03)	(0.03)
Generations	−0.05	0.025	0.04	−0.00	0.01	0.02	0.02	0.02
	(0.04)	(0.04)	(0.04)	(0.04)	(0.01)	(0.01)	(0.01)	(0.01)

Region: Kyungsang	0.07	0.09	0.02	0.04	0.00	0.01	−0.00	−0.00
	(0.12)	(0.12)	(0.12)	(0.12)	(0.04)	(0.04)	(0.04)	(0.04)
Region: Jeolla	0.19	0.11	0.09	0.12	0.03	0.03	0.03	0.03
	(0.17)	(0.17)	(0.17)	(0.17)	(0.05)	(0.05)	(0.05)	(0.05)
Constant					−0.35*	−0.43**	−0.42**	−0.44**
					(0.14)	(0.14)	(0.14)	(0.14)
Observations	1,832	1,832	1,832	1,832	1,832	1,832	1,832	1,832
Adj. R-squared	0.340	0.360	0.350	0.380	0.0204	0.0328	0.0402	0.0408

Note: Robust standard errors in parentheses
* $p < 0.05$, ** $p < 0.01$, *** $p < 0.001$.

deviations for both waves are 0.75 and 0.82, the level of government trust declined by an average of 0.44 at the aggregate level.

Overall, these results suggest that Korean citizens evaluate government performance on salient issues and adjust levels of political trust at the individual level. In particular, they positively assessed the government's response to COVID-19, which sustained their confidence in the government. On the other hand, their negative evaluation of government policies on real estate led to a significant decline in political trust. Citizens' evaluations of the economy had mixed effects on government trust and its changes. Besides these individual-level effects, government trust substantially waned between the two waves at the aggregate level.

Furthermore, it is notable that the decline in government trust is primarily evident among those politically unaffiliated in Step 2. Except for the variable of performance evaluation of real estate, no other variables are related to changes in government trust. These results demonstrate that government performance is a major source of Korea's political dynamics, with politically unaffiliated citizens forming a swing force behind the dynamic. When these two findings are combined, it is clear that Korean citizens consider substantial government performance to be a key factor when revising political trust (Choi and Woo, 2016; Wang, 2016).

On April 7, 2021, three weeks after the second wave of the panel survey, the ruling party was defeated in the by-elections for the Seoul and Pusan metropolitan mayors. These by-elections were unique because both former mayors of Seoul and Pusan, affiliated with the ruling Democratic Party, stepped down due to sexual scandals. Nonetheless, the Moon Jae-in government was unprepared for the post-pandemic situation and failed to address salient issues other than COVID-19. This contributed to the lame-duck period of the Moon Jae-in government, leading to significant losses for the Democratic Party.

During the five years of the Moon Jae-in government, real estate and apartment prices continued to rise, disappointing middle- and lower-class supporters and irritating upper-class voters. Moreover, the politically unaffiliated began to view the ruling Democratic party as incapable and incompetent in addressing those salient issues such as the economy and real estate. This perception grew because the ruling party held both legislative and executive power after the legislative elections in April 2020. This is the political paradox of Korea's success against COVID-19: The early success against the pandemic reduced public concerns and fear, causing Korean citizens to shift their focus to other pressing issues. The Moon Jae-in government missed the opportunity to recover political trust among Korean citizens afterward. In other words, the short-term success against COVID-19 failed to translate into long-term political success. In the end, the ruling Democratic Party lost the next presidential election in March 2022.

Conclusion: Dynamic but Enduring State-Society Relations of Korea

This chapter attempted to shed light on Korean society and politics during the first year of the COVID-19 pandemic. We examined why the early success of the Moon Jae-in government in combating COVID-19 did not lead to long-term political success. To address this central question, we focused on government trust and its change. Political trust is vital in democracy because it changes over time, making democratic politics dynamic and accountable. Hence, we analyzed government trust and traced how Korea's response to COVID-19 affected political trust.

Analytically, we used a two-wave panel survey. The first wave was conducted in the early summer of 2020 when the Moon Jae-in government successfully contained the widespread transmission of COVID-19. The second wave was in the spring of 2021 when the government began to experience a lame-duck period. Through this panel survey, we identified two main findings. First, Korea's early response to COVID-19 was notably successful, leading to political consequences such as high government trust (60%) and a landslide victory for the ruling party in the 2020 legislative elections. Korea succeeded against COVID-19 for two reasons. One was that Korea had learned from the failure of the 2015 MERS response, maintaining medical and preventive preparedness even after MERS ended. Koreans became accustomed to using hand sanitizer and masks during MERS, and the government implemented contact tracing and quarantine from 2015 to 2019, even after MERS had subsided. This extensive medical preparedness worked well in the early period of the COVID-19 pandemic. Since MERS and COVID-19 are coronavirus variants causing respiratory problems, the outbreak of COVID-19 could be seen as an extension of MERS. The second reason was that the failure of the MERS response caused political damage to the former Park Geun-hye government, leading the Moon Jae-in government to implement a consistent statewide response to COVID-19 and other natural disasters. This approach deserves recognition.

Second, government trust fell by 14% between the first and second waves of the panel survey. This indicates that about one-third of those who trusted the government in the first wave switched to distrust in the second wave. We proposed that citizens evaluate government performance across various salient issues, with salience varying among them. We demonstrated that whereas the successful response to COVID-19 sustained government trust, the unsuccessful response to real estate led to political distrust. The early success against COVID-19 alleviated public fear and concern, allowing Koreans to focus on other relevant issues such as real estate and the economy. Negative performance evaluation on these two issues caused a decline in government trust, from which the Moon Jae-in government could not recover. This effect was particularly evident among political independents. These results suggest that government performance is a primary factor in Korea's political dynamics, with political independents playing a key role in driving these dynamics.

What do these analytical results imply for Korean politics and society? They suggest that Korean citizens prioritize substantive performance on relevant issues when adjusting their political trust. This aligns with prior studies indicating that East Asian people value tangible results more than procedural justice (Choi and Woo, 2016; Wang, 2016). These results also show that democratic accountability functions in Korea, as Korean citizens support or punish leaders based on their performance. However, they imply that Korean politics is dynamic but unstable, given that sudden fluctuations in government trust do not necessarily lead to political success and failure. In terms of state-society relations, prominent scholars of Korean politics identify strong state, contentious society, and unstable politics (Cho et al., 2019; Henderson, 1968; S. Kim, 2000). Our research concludes that Korea's primary features of state-society relations persisted, rather than changed, during and after the COVID-19 pandemic.

Acknowledgment

This work was supported by the Ministry of Education of the Republic of Korea and the National Research Foundation of Korea (NRF-2022S1A5A2A01048366).

References

Aassve, Arnstein, Tommaso Capezzone, Nicolò Cavalli, Pierluigi Conzo, and Chen Peng. 2024. Social and political trust diverge during a crisis. *Scientific Reports* 14(1): 331.

Bækgaard, Martin, Jake Christensen, Jan K. Madsen, and Sass Mikkelsen Kim. 2020. Rallying around the flag in times of COVID-19: Societal lockdown and trust in democratic institutions. *Journal of Behavioral Public Administration* 3(2): 1–12.

Bartels, Larry M. 1996. Uninformed votes: Information effects in presidential elections. *American Journal of Political Science* 40(1): 194–230.

Belchior, Ana Maria, and Conceição Pequito Teixeira. 2023. Determinants of political trust during the early months of the COVID-19 pandemic: Putting policy performance into evidence. *Political Studies Review* 21(1): 82–98.

Beschel, Robert. 2021. *Policy and Institutional Response to COVID-19 in the Middle East and North Africa.* Brooking Institute Report. www.brookings.edu/articles/policy-and-institutional-responses-to-covid-19-in-the-middle-east-and-north-africa-egypt/

Bol, Damien, Marco Giani, Andre Blais, and Peter John Loewen. 2020. The effect of COVID-19 lockdowns on political support: Some good news for democracy? *European Journal of Political Research* 60(2): 497–505.

Bourgeois, Laura French, Allison Harell, and Laura B. Stephenson. 2020. To follow or not to follow: Social norms and civic duty during a pandemic. *Canadian Journal of Political Science* 53(2): 273–278.

Carlin, Ryan E., Gregory J. Love, and Elizabeth J. Zechmeister. 2014. Trust shaken: earthquake damage, state capacity, and interpersonal trust in comparative perspective. *Comparative Politics* 46(4): 419–453.

Chanley, Virginia A. 2002. Trust in government in the aftermath of 9/11: Determinants and consequences. *Political Psychology* 23(3): 469–483.

Chanley, Virginia A., Thomas J. Rudolph, and Wendy M. Rahn. 2000. The origins and consequences of public trust in government: A time series analysis. *Public Opinion Quarterly* 64(3): 239–256.

Cho, Youngho. 2019. MERS disaster and declining trust in government under the Park Geun-hye Administration. *Journal of Korean Politics* 28(2): 167–193.

Cho, Youngho, Mi-son Kim, and Yong Cheol Kim. 2019. Cultural foundation of contentious democracy. *Asian Survey* 59(2): 272–294.

Choi, Eunjung, and Jongseok Woo. 2016. The origins of political trust in East Asian democracies: Psychological, cultural, and institutional arguments. *Japanese Journal of Political Science* 17(3): 410–426.

Chung, Tae-Il. 2016. The critical study on the election revolution in the 20th National Assembly election. *The Institute for Northeast Asia Research* 31(2): 5–32.

Citrin, Jack, and Laura Stoker. 2018. Political trust in a cynical age. *Annual Review of Political Science* 21: 49–70.

Dahl, Robert. 1971. *Polyarchy: Participation and Opposition*. New Haven, CT: Yale University Press.

Gallup Korea. 2020. Daily Opinion No. 354 (3rd Week of May 2019). Gallup Korea. www.gallup.co.kr/gallupdb/reportContent.asp?seqNo=1013.

Gallup Korea. 2021. Daily Opinion No. 440 (3rd Week of March 2021). Gallup Korea. www.gallup.co.kr/gallupdb/reportContent.asp?seqNo=1187.

Healy, Andrew, and Neil Malhotra. 2009. Myopic voters and natural disaster policy. *American Political Science Review* 103(3): 387–406.

Healy, Andrew, and Neil Malhotra. 2013. Retrospective voting reconsidered. *Annual Review of Political Science* 16: 285–306.

Henderson, Gregory, 1968. *Korea, the Politics of the Vortex*. Cambridge, MA: Harvard University Press.

Hetherington, Marc J. 1998. The political relevance of political trust. *American Political Science Review* 92(4): 791–808.

Hetherington, Marc J., and Thomas J. Rudolph. 2015. *Why Washington Won't Work: Polarization, Political Trust, and the Governing Crisis*. Chicago, IL: University of Chicago Press.

James, Sarah, Caroline Tervo, and Theda Skocpol. 2022. Institutional capacities, partisan divisions, and federal tensions in US responses to the COVID-19 pandemic. *RSF: The Russell Sage Foundation Journal of the Social Sciences* 8(8): 154–180.

Ji, Chengyuan, Junyan Jiang, and Yujin Zhang. 2024. Political trust and government performance in the time of COVID-19. *World Development* 176: 106499.

Kallemose, Thomas, John W. Kirk, Elinor K. Karlsson, Ida Seing, Nina Thórný Stefánsdóttir, Karsten Vrangbæk, Ove Andersen, and Per Nilsen. 2023. Political trust in the handling of the COVID-19 pandemic: A survey in Denmark and Sweden. *BMC Global and Public Health* 1(1): 1–10.

Kang, JaHyun, Yun Young Jang, JinHwa Kim, Si-Hyeon Han, Ki Rog Lee, Mukju Kim, and Joong Sik Eom. 2020. South Korea's responses to stop the COVID-19 pandemic. *American Journal of Infection Control* 48(9): 1080–1086.

Kim, June-Ho, Julia Ah-Reum An, SeungJu Jackie Oh, Juhwan Oh, and Jong-Koo Lee. 2020. Emerging COVID-19 success story: South Korea learned the lessons of MERS. Published online at OurWorldInData.org. https://ourworldindata.org/covid-exemplar-south-korea.

Kim, Sunhyuk. 2000. *The Politics of Democratization in Korea: The Role of Civil Society*. Pittsburgh, PA: University of Pittsburgh Press.

Korea Financial Investment Association. 2022. *Comparison of Household Financial Assets in Major Countries for 2022*. International Survey Department. www.kofia.or.kr/brd/m_48/down.do?brd_id=www_research&seq=213&data_tp=A&file_seq=1.

Kwon, Hee-rim. 2021. During Moon's 4-Year Term, Seoul Apartment Prices Doubled. *The JoongAng* (June 24, 2021). www.joongang.co.kr/article/24089598.

Lim, Soo, and Minji Sohn. 2023. How to cope with emerging viral diseases: Lessons from South Korea's strategy for COVID-19, and collateral damage to cardiometabolic health. *The Lancet Regional Health–Western Pacific* 30: 100581.

Miller, Arthur H. 1974. Political issues and trust in government: 1964–1970. *American Political Science Review* 68(3): 951–972.

Moon, M. Jae. 2020. Fighting COVID-19 with agility, transparency, and participation: Wicked policy problems and new governance challenges. *Public Administration Review* 80(4): 651–656.

Moon, M. Jae, Kohei Suzuki, Tae In Park, and Kentaro Sakuwa. 2021. A comparative study of COVID-19 responses in South Korea and Japan: Political nexus triad and policy responses. *International Review of Administrative Sciences* 87(3): 651–671.

OECD. 2023. *Ready for the Next Crisis? Investing in Health System Resilience*. OECD Health Policy Studies.

Our World in Data. 2023. South Korea: Coronavirus Pandemic Country Profile. Published online at OurWorldInData.org. https://ourworldindata.org/coronavirus/country/south-korea

Park, June, and Eunbin Chung. 2021. Learning from past pandemic governance: Early response and public-private partnerships in testing of COVID-19 in South Korea. *World Development* 137: 105198.

Parsons, Sam, and Richard D. Wiggins. 2020. *Trust in Government and Others during the COVID-19 Pandemic—Initial Findings from the COVID-19 Survey in Five National Longitudinal Studies*. London: UCL Centre for Longitudinal Studies.

Pharr, Susan J., and Robert D Putnam. 2000. *Disaffected Democracies: What's Troubling the Trilateral Countries?* Princeton, NJ: Princeton University Press.

Popkin, Samuel L. 1991. *The Reasoning Voter: Communication and Persuasion in Presidential Campaigns*. Chicago, IL: University of Chicago Press.

Putnam, Robert D. 1993. The prosperous community. *The American Prospect* 4(13): 35–42.

Rieger, Marc Oliver, and Mei Wang. 2022. Trust in government actions during the COVID-19 crisis. *Social Indicators Research* 159(3): 967–989.

Roh, Gi-Woo, Jungsub Shin, and Youngho Cho. 2021. The effects of citizens' policy evaluation on government trust. *The Institute for Far Eastern Studies* 1: 297–329.

Schraff, Dominik. 2021. Political trust during the Covid-19 pandemic: Rally around the flag or lockdown effects? *European Journal of Political Research* 60(4): 1007–1017.

Su, Zhenhua, Shan Su, and Qian Zhou. 2021. Government trust in a time of crisis. *China Review* 21(2): 87–116.

Suhay, Elizabeth, Aparna Soni, Claudia Persico, and Dave E. Marcotte. 2022. Americans' trust in government and health behaviors during the COVID-19 pandemic. *RSF: The Russell Sage Foundation Journal of the Social Sciences* 8(8): 221–244.

Van der Meer, Tom, and Armen Hakhverdian. 2017. Political trust as the evaluation of process and performance: A cross-national study of 42 European countries. *Political Studies* 65(1): 81–102.

Van der Meer, Tom, Eefje Steenvoorden, and Ebe Ouattara. 2023. Fear and the COVID-19 rally round the flag: A panel study on political trust. *West European Politics* 46(6): 1089–1105.

Wang, Ching-Hsing. 2016. Government performance, corruption, and political trust in East Asia. *Social Science Quarterly* 97(2): 211–231.

Zaller, John. 1992. *The Nature and Origins of Mass Opinion*. Cambridge, UK: Cambridge University Press.

4 Chinese Citizens' Voices in the Shadow of COVID-19

Yida Zhai

Introduction

The management strategies and responses to the COVID-19 pandemic vary by country and are contingent on each nation's political system and culture. Since the initial outbreak in 2019, China implemented stringent measures, including lockdowns and extended quarantine, and has promoted a large-scale vaccination campaign. Although most countries worldwide gradually returned to normal life and lifted their COVID-19 countermeasures, China maintained its zero-COVID policy, that is, the nation's refusal to coexist with the virus and its prioritization of zero infections over economic development and ordinary people's regular lives (Zhai, 2023). The zero-COVID policy represents the state's formidable intervention to control and prevent the worsening of the outbreak. Experts stated that this policy should be highly evaluated, as it has significantly reduced infections and deaths compared to situations where such a policy has not been adopted (Chen and Chen,2022; Zhang et al., 2022). The Chinese government is proud of its policy and claims that it is scientific and effective and stands the test of time.

In China's political system, upward accountability motivates local government officials to strictly implement the national government's policy on some occasions. Under the zero-COVID policy, local government officials risk dismissal if there is viral spread in their region. More transmissible COVID-19 variants have created great difficulty in terms of the speedy detection of new infection cases and the identification of the close contacts of affected persons, as well as the imposition of effective quarantine and isolation. Fear of being accused of irresponsibility motivates officials' excessive use of lockdowns to contain the viral spread. Keng et al. (2024) state that the zero-COVID policy was related to Xi's third term as the CCP general secretary. The government further tightened the control measures before the 20th Party Congress. From late August 2022 until the policy was abandoned, more than 74 cities imposed full or partial lockdowns which impacted more than 313 million people (Gan and Deng, 2022).Although the zero-COVID policy caused significant disruption to people's daily lives, the policy did not face widespread opposition during the first two years of the pandemic. While those directly affected by lockdowns expressed dissatisfaction with the policy (Han and Zhai, 2024b; Gan, 2022; Zhai and Han, 2024), people in other regions supported

DOI: 10.4324/9781003495239-5

the stringent measures, as they helped prevent the spread of the virus to their cities. However, the emergence of the Omicron variant in 2022 made it increasingly difficult to sustain the zero-COVID policy, and local governments were forced to implement lockdowns. As more cities imposed lockdowns, a growing number of Chinese people began to experience the negative impacts of the policy and acknowledged its shortcomings. Long-lasting restrictions caused a decline in their support for the government (Guan et al., 2024; Zeng, 2024; Zhai, 2023). In November 2022, the Chinese people took to the streets to protest COVID-19 restrictions in more than 20 cities, including Beijing, Nanjing, Wuhan, Chongqing, Chengdu, Guangzhou, and Shanghai (Gan and Wang, 2022).

However, it goes too far to argue that a large proportion of Chinese people were involved in the protests. The protests had a greater impact abroad than domestically. The Western media overstated the resistance of a few young people. Due to information censorship, many ordinary Chinese citizens were unaware of the protests that took place at the end of 2022. Furthermore, these protests did not indicate a widespread intent to overthrow China's one-party system. Chinese people tolerated the sufferings from the subsequent lifting of the zero-COVID policy and continued to maintain obedience to authority. The protests at the end of 2022 cannot deny the fact that the Chinese government had successfully sustained its stringent approach for two and a half years, which was impossible in other parts of the world. By contrast, American and European residents have organized rallies to protest against local COVID-19 countermeasures (Crow and Waldmeir, 2020; Iddiols and Shelley, 2021). Although China has an authoritarian political system, the implementation of the zero-COVID policy does not completely depend on oppressive and violent methods. Chinese citizens' willingness to comply with the policy is indispensable. Some citizens have offered various justifications for the policy and defended the government's failures in the process of combating the pandemic.

Chinese citizens' voices provide important insights into understanding the endurance of China's strategies for tackling COVID-19. Previous studies found that Chinese people positively evaluated their country's response to the pandemic and showed considerable tolerance for the lockdown policy prior to the spread of the Omicron variant (Guan et al., 2024; Wu et al., 2021; Zhai, 2024). Adopting a bottom-up approach allows us to explore the reasons the apparently unwelcome policy can be maintained. This chapter analyzes Chinese citizens' policy preference regarding the (non-)restriction of freedoms, their perceptions of where the responsibility for infection prevention and control lies, and their willingness to comply with the state's anti-COVID-19 policy.

Moreover, the zero-COVID policy has severely damaged the economy, which has, in turn, worsened Chinese people's economic lives. Economic hardship may increase citizens' support for the expansion of the state's intervention in economic activities. Meanwhile, social capital provides resources and support for people amid economic hardship. Consequently, people with greater social capital may resist the expansion of the state's economic intervention. Hence, this chapter also examines Chinese citizens' attitudes toward the expansion of the state's economic role in the post-pandemic era, as well as the effects of economic hardship and social capital on these attitudes. The results of the analysis illustrate the mass psychological bases of China's anti-COVID-19 policies and identify the changing relationship between Chinese citizens and the state in the post-pandemic era.

Support for the State's Restriction of Individual Freedoms

Understanding Tolerance for the Restriction of Freedom

There exists a trade-off between speedy control of the pandemic and the maintenance of citizens' freedoms. To contain the spread of the virus, strict measures must be adopted, and freedoms are subject to violation. In February 2020, an expert from Shanghai Mental Health Center appealed to people to suppress their natural instinct to exercise their personal freedom and comply with the state's anti-COVID-19 measures. The zero-COVID policy aims to contain the outbreak by closing cross-infection transmission routes, which entails the strict restriction of people's daily activities and freedoms. Indeed, people have debated such restrictions. Some view restricting people's mobility and freedom to have social gatherings as well as imposing lockdowns and related policies as unnecessary. In their minds, restricting freedom is unacceptable, even to prevent infection. People understandably treasure their freedom. Opposition to anti-COVID-19 measures on these grounds challenges the government. The Chinese government can more easily enforce its zero-COVID policy if citizens prioritize infection control over their freedom.

The existing literature has examined several of the Chinese government's strategies to induce citizens' tolerance for the restriction of their freedom during the pandemic. First, China demonized the virus to terrify Chinese people and obtain support for strict anti-COVID-19 measures. Uncertainty makes individuals prone to comply with powerful leadership (Hogg, 2005, 2007). During the pandemic, the looming external threat promoted support for the lockdown policy (Zhai, 2024). Through censorship and propaganda, the state-run media circulated information about the large number of infections and deaths in other countries that failed to impose strict measures. The Chinese government is obsessed with the pursuit of zero infection, and it persuades people to believe in the necessity of restricted freedom for the sake of disease control.

Second, China used the pandemic as an instrument to demonstrate the superiority of its political system, which has an advantage in terms of its ability to control the viral spread (Xi, 2020). China politicized the contrast between its zero-COVID policy and Western countries' policy of coexistence with the virus as a competition between political systems, national power, and civilizations (Shen, 2022). Tolerance for the restriction of freedom under the zero-COVID policy is a matter of political correctness in the Chinese context. The authorities warned that the government would resolutely fight against anyone who questioned or negated the zero-COVID policy (Xinhua News Agency, 2022). Individual freedoms are trivial compared to the state's determination to achieve zero infection. The contrast with Western countries' approach coupled with nationalism motivated the Chinese people to tolerate the restriction of their freedom to achieve the national zero infection goal.

Unlike previous research, this chapter positions political culture as a driver of Chinese citizens' tolerance for the state's restriction of their freedom. Political culture theory emphasizes the psycho-cultural dimension of politics, such as citizens' perceptions and evaluation of government policies and their value orientation to politics (Almond and Verba, 1963; Inglehart and Welzel, 2005; Shi, 2014). Confucianism has a longstanding influence in China; it penetrates Chinese people's familial, social, and political relations and shapes their behavior (Fetzer and Soper, 2010; Yao, 2000). Since the Han Dynasty, the literate elite allied with the monarchy and distorted authentic Confucian scholarship to create state ideology (Liu, 1996; Wright, 1975: vii). This politicized Confucianism bred a paternalist political culture, which serves rulers' interests and has become dominant in Chinese society. Paternalist political culture highlights a two-sided relationship between individuals and the state (Hahm, 2004). On the one hand, the people owe their obedience to the state. On the other hand, the state is responsible for taking care of the people and protecting their welfare. Individual autonomy and self-reliance are discouraged in paternalist political culture. Empirical studies have shown that the Chinese public has a high level of obedience to the authorities (Zhai, 2017, 2022).

In addition, China saw the importation of liberal culture as of the end of the 19th century. In the early 20th century, "progressive" intellectuals attempted to reform China by introducing liberal culture and advocating for social transformation through liberalization and democratization. Liberalism competed with nationalism, statism, and communism in China but never managed to dominate other thought in the 20th century. After the Cultural Revolution, there came a short liberal cultural boom during the 1980s, but it could not persist and was interrupted after the 1989 Tiananmen Square protests. Given that liberal culture stresses individual autonomy, sensitivity to the state's power, and the guarantee of civil and political liberties, Chinese rulers dislike it, and they spare no effort in attempting to control and eliminate its influence. Despite authoritarian suppression, globalization and economic and cultural exchanges with foreign countries have made isolating China from the influence of liberal culture impossible. China's political culture is also subject to change under t Western influence (Chu and Yu, 1993; Hua, 2001). In present-day Chinese society, authoritarian paternalist values and liberal values coexist. Chinese society is polarized due to stance divisions in debates over various public issues along the boundary of these two political and cultural camps.

Amid the pandemic, the public's concerns about infection rise, but their attribution of the responsibility for infection prevention and control affects their policy preference. Political culture influences whether people attribute responsibility to the state or to individuals. Specifically, liberal and paternalist values shape Chinese citizens' perceptions of where the responsibility for infection prevention and control lies. Liberal values stress individual autonomy and promote people's self-attribution of responsibility. In contrast, paternalist values stress people's incapability of addressing a public health emergency such as COVID-19 and promote people's attribution of that responsibility to the state. In the paternalist belief system, citizens' perceptions of their incapability and incompetency and the desire for the state's benevolent protection are two sides of the same coin. As previously mentioned, political culture is a strong determinant of whether people attribute the responsibility for infection prevention and control to the state or to the individual. Attribution of responsibility is significant because it suggests whether governments will be under fire in the event that infections and deaths rise. Hence, studying how citizens attribute responsibility will deepen our knowledge of the citizen-state relationship in China.

This chapter examined the relationship between anti-COVID-19 policy preference and attribution of the responsibility for infection prevention and control. Table 4.1 presents the results of a contingency table analysis with two categorical variables: policy preference (opposition to the restriction of freedom, neutral, and support for the restriction of freedom) and attribution of responsibility (the individual's responsibility, neutral, and the state's responsibility). The results show that Chinese citizens' anti-COVID-19 policy preference was not independent of their attribution of the responsibility for infection prevention and control, $\chi^2 = 116.678$, $p < 0.001$. People who believed in individual responsibility for infection prevention tended to oppose anti-COVID-19 measures entailing the restriction of individual freedom, while those who believed the state was responsible for controlling infection were more likely to support the restriction of freedom.

Paternalist political culture encourages citizens' obedience to and dependence on the state. According to the results, Chinese people who adhered to a paternalist citizen-state relationship tended to attribute the responsibility for infection prevention and control to the state rather than to themselves. The survey data demonstrate that they showed high levels of understanding of the zero-COVID policy and had a higher tolerance for the state's restriction of individual freedoms.

Table 4.1 Variations in policy preference across types of responsibility attribution

		Attitudes toward restriction on freedom			
		Opposition	*Neutral*	*Support*	*Total*
Attribution of the responsibility for infection prevention and control	Individual responsibility	104 (34.21%)	47 (15.46%)	153 (50.33%)	304 (30.4%)
	Neutral	37 (15.95%)	36 (15.52%)	159 (68.53%)	232 (23.20%)
	The state's responsibility	32 (6.90%)	43 (9.27%)	389 (83.84%)	464 (46.40%)
	Total	173 (17.30%)	126 (12.60%)	701 (70.10%)	1000 (100%)

Willingness to Comply with Anti-COVID-19 Policies

A Sub-National Perspective

China has a vast territory, and the significant regional differences cannot be neglected. Since the 1980s, China has opted for an imbalanced development strategy. Chinese political leaders prioritized prosperity in the coastal region and recruited prosperous residents in that area to help others toward achieving common prosperity. Specifically, the state prioritized modernization of the eastern region through substantial financial support and favorable policies. This unbalanced development policy has stimulated China's economic growth but created tremendous gaps in terms of socioeconomic levels and household living standards across regions (Li et al., 2017). For instance, the eastern region's per capita gross domestic product (GDP) is threefold larger than that of the western region. People in economically less developed regions have expressed resentment toward the national government's imbalanced development strategy. Regional economic disparities have also generated various social problems, such as increasing geographic prejudice among regions. Chinese citizens' evaluations of the government's policy performance also vary across regions. The sub-national perspective is valuable for recognizing regional differences within China.

With a few exceptions, most studies on public opinion in China treated the country as a homogeneous entity and analyzed it as a whole. This chapter adopts a sub-national perspective to examine regional variations in public opinion within China. Based on specific research themes, there are different methods for dividing China into regions. Talhelm et al. (2014) categorized China into northern and southern regions using the Yangtze River as a divider. Lewis-Beck et al. (2014) divided China into eight regions: northeast, north, east, central, northwest, southwest, and municipal regions. Dickson et al. (2017) categorized coastal, northeast, and central regions. Zhai (2021) employed a three-region division: eastern, central, and western. Conventionally, the National Bureau of Statistics of China categorized the country into the eastern, central, and western regions, according to their respective economic development levels, but this approach was replaced by a four-region categorization as of 2011. Adhering to this new classification, the present study divided the country into the eastern, central, western, and northeast regions. In our survey, respondents were asked to indicate the extent of their willingness to comply with the state's anti-COVID-19 policy on a five-point scale. This chapter examines differences in Chinese citizens' policy compliance across the four abovementioned regions.

Analysis of variance (ANOVA) shows a significant effect of region on Chinese people's willingness to comply with anti-COVID-19 policies, F (3, 996) = 4.02, p = .007, $\eta_p^2 = 0.012$. The results of post-hoc analyses using Scheffe's test indicate significantly lower policy compliance in the western region (M = 4.096, SD = 0.887) than in the eastern region (M = 4.303, SD = 0.763), p = 0.025. In addition, policy compliance in the western region was weakly significantly lower than that in the northeastern region (M = 4.370, SD = 0.720), p = 0.054. The results demonstrate regional gaps in Chinese people's tendency to comply with the state's anti-COVID-19 policy. The western region is the least economically developed in China, and its residents were less satisfied with the government's performance. Consequently, they had low levels of policy compliance.

The Relationship between Policy Preference and Policy Compliance

People's willingness to comply with a certain policy is linked to their policy preference. Although the zero-COVID policy resulted in indefinite isolation, damaged the economy, and created inconvenience in people's daily lives, some people support it and believe that it is justifiable because zero tolerance for the virus can save more lives. Conversely, others oppose the policy because it violates individual freedoms and liberties. People's preference for different policies reveals their fundamental attitudes. If an individual dislikes a certain policy, there is a strong possibility that they will resist it. Moreover, people's perceptions of where the responsibility for infection prevention and control lies may also be related to their willingness to comply with the state's anti-COVID-19 policy. The successful implementation of any policy depends on citizens' compliance. Tangible deterrence measures cannot ensure people's voluntary adherence to a state policy. Previous studies investigated normative and instrumental factors as motivations for compliance (Gao and Zhao, 2017; Martín et al., 2012; Yagil, 1998). Given that policy preference and perceptions of responsibility play important roles in willingness to comply with related policies, this chapter aims to examine whether people's policy preference regarding freedom and the attribution of the responsibility for infection prevention and control contribute to (non-)compliance with the state's anti-COVID-19 measures.

First, this study investigated the Chinese people's willingness to comply with the state's anti-COVID-19 policy. According to the survey results, the majority of Chinese people (86.70%) were willing to comply with the policy, while 8% were neutral, and 5.3% were non-compliant. Multivariate regression analysis was performed to examine the relationships between demographic attributes, policy preference, and the attribution of the responsibility for infection prevention and control and willingness to comply with the state's anti-COVID-19 policy. The following demographic variables were considered: age, gender, education level, income, area of residence (rural vs. urban), and subjective social class (upper, upper middle, lower middle, working, and lower). Due to regional variations, Chinese people's policy compliance was investigated in the eastern, central, western, and northeastern regions, respectively. Figure 4.1 presents the results.

In the eastern region, support for the restriction of freedom positively predicted people's willingness to comply with the state's anti-COVID-19 policy ($b = 0.389$, $p < 0.001$). However, attribution of the responsibility for infection prevention and control and respondents' other demographic attributes were not significantly associated with policy compliance.

In the central region, support for the restriction of freedom positively predicted willingness to comply with the state's policy ($b = 0.316$, $p < .001$), while

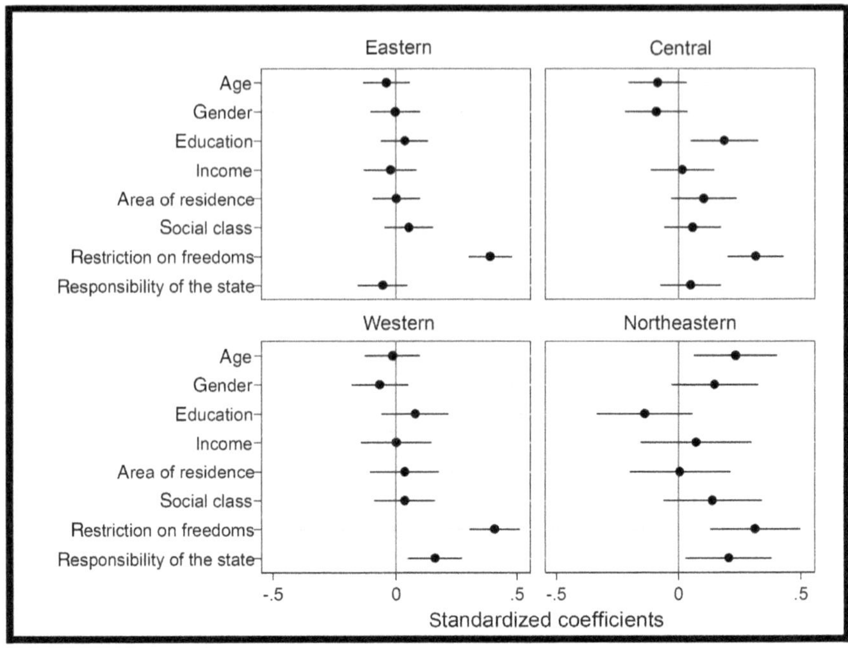

Figure 4.1 Predicting people's willingness to comply with anti-COVID-19 policies.

attribution of the responsibility for infection prevention and control was not significantly associated with policy compliance. Regarding respondents' demographic characteristics, people with higher education levels tended to have high degrees of policy compliance (b = 0.188, p = 0.011). The effects of other demographic variables were not significant.

In the western region, both support for the restriction of freedom during the pandemic and perceiving infection prevention and control as the state's responsibility positively predicted willingness to comply with the state's policy (b = 0.408, p < 0.001; b = 0.162, p = 0.006). Demographic attributes were not significantly associated with policy compliance.

In the northeastern region, support for the restriction of freedom and attributing the responsibility for infection prevention and control to the state positively predicted willingness to comply with the state's policy (b = 0.314, p = 0.003; b = 0.206, p = 0.035). Older generations also tended to have high levels of policy compliance (b = 0.233, p = 0.016). Other demographic attributes were not significantly associated with willingness to comply with the state's anti-COVID-19 policy.

Generally, a policy preference skewed toward the restriction of freedom during the pandemic resulted in high compliance with the state's anti-COVID-19 policy in all four regions. The results indicate that the relationship between policy preference and policy compliance was consistent and universal in every region of China. Specifically, people who favor the restriction of individual freedoms for the sake of infection prevention and control amid the pandemic would be willing to comply with the zero-COVID policy in China, while those who prioritize individual freedoms would resist the policy.

However, the attribution of the responsibility for infection prevention and control to the state facilitated policy compliance in the western and northeastern regions. The results indicate that paternalist culture, which encourages deference to and dependence on the state, is more influential in these two regions. Its influence is weaker in the eastern and central regions partially because of the high levels of modernization there. Adherence to paternalist culture was lower among residents of the eastern and central regions; hence, the perception of infection prevention and control as the state's responsibility failed to motivate those people to support the state's stringent anti-COVID-19 policy. The sub-national perspective and the political culture approach have provided new insights into understanding Chinese people's support for the zero-COVID policy.

Favorable Attitudes toward the State's Role in the Economy

Expectations of the State's Expanded Economic Role

The degree to which the state intervenes in economic activities varies by country. In some countries, the state plays a considerable role in the economy, such as intervening in industrial investment and devising state-led development plans. In other countries, the state refrains from intervening in the economy, which primarily depends on private capitalism. Discussion of the state's economic role should not be isolated from a country's contextual situation.

In the Mao era, China had a planned economy, in which a centralized planning system organized and managed production, distribution, and consumption throughout the country. This economic model was adopted from the Soviet Union and widely practiced in other socialist countries. In a planned economy, the state replaces the market and plays a dominant role in economic activities. After socialist reform in China in 1956, the operation of private firms was disallowed, and the state established numerous state-owned enterprises that were characterized by low efficiency because they could extract subsidies or loans from the government and banks without a fixed budget. Kornai (1980) called this phenomenon the soft budget constraint syndrome. Despite their low efficiency, state-owned enterprises constituted an important unit in Chinese urban society. They were not only economic organizations but also suppliers of social welfare. It was state-owned enterprises that built hospitals, schools, and sports and entertainment facilities. Hence, they were described as "small society." Furthermore, through state-owned enterprises, the state organized skills training for workers, controlled income distribution, managed employment, provided social welfare, and invested in industry.

China's economic reform entailed a transition from a planned economy to a market-oriented economy, which saw the state retreat from some areas of various economic fields. This transition stimulated rapid national economic growth, and ordinary people's living standards improved substantially. In fact, China has become the world's second-largest economy. However, among its people, the income gap has widened significantly. China changed from an egalitarian society in the Mao period to an unequal society after the 1980s. As a macro indicator of economic inequality, China's Gini coefficient reached a range of 0.53 to 0.55 and ranked among the highest in the world (Xie and Zhou, 2014). Chinese people's critical attitudes toward income inequality generate public distrust in the government (Lei, 2020; Zhou and Jin, 2018).

Economic reform has had a two-fold impact on Chinese people's everyday lives. On the one hand, people's efforts are rewarded, and those who contribute more have a high income. This change would have been unimaginable in the Mao era when poverty was universal, but income remained equal across society. On the other hand, presently, individuals who do not have an advantage in terms of market competition have a low income. Meritocracy further justifies their disadvantaged position through the discourse on incapability and incompetence. Such people feel that they do not benefit from the economic reform and are even nostalgic for the Maoist era.

Economic hardship often boosts the public's support for the state's assumption of a significant role in the economy. Amid crises, the government expands its power for the sake of emergency response and reinforces authoritarian control over society (Woods et al., 2020; Zhai, 2023). In the Chinese context, economic crisis usually evokes citizens' criticism of market-oriented reform; meanwhile, appeals for the state's intervention in the economy rise. The COVID-19 pandemic has resulted in the economic downturn in China (Liu, 2021; Zhao et al., 2021), and the zero-COVID policy inflicted further damage on the nation's economy. Lockdowns and other strict countermeasures have triggered factory closures, broken supply chains, and increased unemployment. According to the survey results, 50.40% of respondents reported a decreased income.

As previously stated, a sub-national perspective is needed to examine regional differences in China. Table 4.2 presents the results of a contingency table analysis of variations in income change during the pandemic across regions. Two categorical variables were used: region (eastern, central, western, and northeastern) and income decline (disagree, neutral, agree). The results show that income change was not independent of region, $\chi^2 = 16.565$, $p = 0.011$. A large proportion of people in the eastern region did not experience income decline, while a large proportion of residents of the northeastern region did.

To examine Chinese citizens' attitudes toward the expansion of the state's economic role, we listed several governmental economic activities and asked respondents to indicate their expectations of the government in the post-pandemic era (see Table 4.3). Creating employment (83.2%) ranked first, followed by the state's other economic roles, namely providing skills training (81.90%), investing in new industries (80.70%), reducing the income gap (77%), and taking care of people who cannot care for themselves (69.8%). The percentage of respondents who

Table 4.2 Variations in income change during the pandemic across different regions

		"During the pandemic, my income has decreased"			
		Disagree	*Neutral*	*Agree*	*Total*
Four regions	Eastern	117 (29.25%)	88 (22.00%)	195 (48.75%)	400 (40%)
	Central	63 (25.20%)	70 (28.00%)	117 (46.80%)	250 (25%)
	Western	65 (26.00%)	60 (24.00%)	125 (50.00%)	250 (25%)
	Northeastern	20 (20.00%)	13 (13.00%)	67 (67.00%)	100 (10%)
	Total	265 (26.50%)	231 (23.10%)	504 (50.40%)	1000 (100%)

Table 4.3 Attitudes toward the state's economic role

	Disagree (%)	*Neutral (%)*	*Agree (%)*
Creating employment	4.7	12.1	83.2
Skills training	6	12.1	81.9
Investing in industrials	4.6	14.7	80.7
Reducing income gap	5.4	17.6	77
Caring people	10.4	19.8	69.8
Taxing the rich	19.8	29.3	50.9

expected the state to tax the rich at a higher rate was the lowest (50.9%), but disagreement on this issue did not exceed one-fifth of all respondents. The results indicate that during the pandemic, Chinese people expected the state to play a greater role in the economy. Nostalgia for the former egalitarian society under the planned economy causes some people to question the market-oriented economy, and they have had reservations all along. Economic hardship has bolstered the Chinese people's support for the state's economic intervention, which justifies the expansion of state power. This tendency has a significant implication in China, where there are less institutional constraints on the state. The government has been exercising its power arbitrarily and frequently infringes on citizens' liberties and rights.

A Social Capital Approach

If economic hardship is positively related to support for greater government intervention in the economy, social capital has a contrary effect. Social capital is an important concept in the contemporary world. It is not only studied in sociology but also widely applied in economics, political science, public health, and other fields. Researchers have not reached a consensus on the definition of social capital. Bourdieu (1986: 248) defines social capital as "the aggregate of the actual or potential resources that are linked to possession of a durable network of more or less institutionalized relationships of mutual acquaintance and recognition." Burt (1992: 9) defines social capital as "friends, colleagues, and more general contacts through whom you receive opportunities to use your financial and human capital." Putnam (1995: 67) defines social capital as the "features of social organization such as networks, norms, and social trust that facilitate coordination and cooperation for mutual benefit." Although the characteristics of social capital are stressed in different manners, most researchers agree that social capital emerges from social interaction and is embedded in interpersonal relationships. Social networks, civic engagement, and social trust are the most frequently used indicators of social capital (Cook, 2005; Mandarano et al., 2010; Putnam, 1993, 1995).

Social capital provides valuable resources for people to manage their lives. In normal times, social capital makes people more competitive in the labor market and helps them achieve career development (Knack and Keefer, 1997; Lin, 2001; Nahapiet and Ghoshal, 1998). In addition, social capital facilitates cooperative action and creates a vibrant civil society (Fukuyama, 2001; Putnam, 1995; Welzel et al., 2005). Amid an emergency, social capital helps people access resources and aid, which supports an effective emergency response and speedy recovery (Cattell, 2001; Han and Zhai, 2024a, 2024b; Sanyal and Routray, 2016). Given that social capital represents resources embedded in social relationships, people with considerable social capital should be more resilient to economic hardship amid the COVID-19 pandemic, and they may not be inclined to support the expansion of the state's role in the economy.

Based on previous studies (Norris, 2002: 137–167; Putnam, 1993, 1995; Subramanian et al., 2001), this chapter operationalized social capital according to its three key components: social networks, civic engagement, and social trust. Social networks were measured by the number of people with whom the respondents had contact on a typical weekday. Civic engagement was measured by the respondents' participation in social organizations, such as environmental, recreational, charitable, religious, and political organizations. Social trust was measured by asking respondents whether they believe that most people can be trusted.

To facilitate comparison, this study standardized the scores for the three components of social capital. Figure 4.2 plots the distribution of social capital in the four regions. ANOVA shows a significant effect of region on social network size, $F\ (3, 996) = 65.51$, $p < 0.001$, $\eta_p^2 = 0.165$. Post-hoc analyses using Scheffe's test indicate that social networks were significantly larger in the eastern region ($M = 0.459$, $SD = 0.968$) than in the central region ($M = -0.362$, $SD = 0.880$), $p < 0.001$, the western region ($M = -0.427$, $SD = 0.817$), $p < 0.001$, and the northeastern region ($M = 0.140$, $SD = 1.014$), $p = 0.021$. Moreover, social networks were significantly larger in the northeastern region than in the central ($p < 0.001$) and western regions ($p < 0.001$).

ANOVA shows regional variations in civic engagement, $F\ (3, 996) = 22.72$, $p < 0.001$, $\eta_p^2 = 0.064$. Post-hoc analyses using Scheffe's test indicate significantly

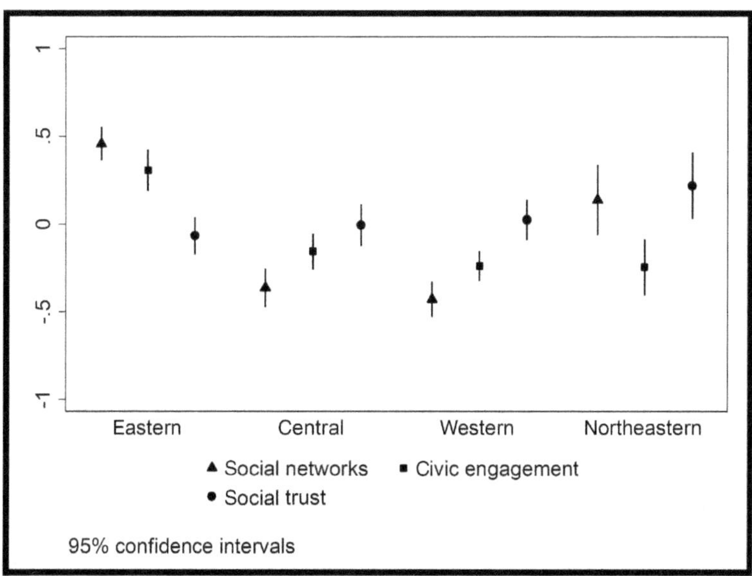

Figure 4.2 Social capital levels in the four regions.

higher civic engagement in the eastern region ($M = 0.307$, $SD = 1.214$) than in the central region ($M = -0.155$, $SD = 0.818$), $p < 0.001$, the western region ($M = -0.238$, $SD = 0.684$), $p < 0.001$, and the northeastern region ($M = -0.245$, $SD = 0.800$), $p < 0.001$. No significant difference was found in the degree of civic engagement between the central, western, and northeastern regions. Additionally, ANOVA also shows that social trust did not vary significantly across the four regions, F (3, 996) = 2.28, $p = 0.078$, $\eta_p^2 = 0.007$.

The aforementioned results indicate significant regional variations in social network size and degree of civic engagement, while social trust remained at a similar level across all four regions. The eastern region is the most economically advanced in China, and this study finds that people's social networks and civic engagement were the strongest there. Previous studies found that social trust can reduce transaction costs and that it affects schooling and the rule of law and facilitates investigation; hence, social trust stimulates economic growth (Beugelsdijk et al., 2004; Bjørnskov, 2012; Whiteley, 2000). As previously stated, China's economic modernization has been unbalanced, and there exists a significant economic gap across regions. However, social trust has remained equal throughout the whole country; hence, a positive relationship between economic development and social trust was not observed at the sub-national level in China.

Moreover, this study created an index for people's expectations of the state's expanded economic role by integrating the six previously mentioned items representing the government's economic activities (see Table 4.3). The scale's

Cronbach's alpha was 0.774, indicating an acceptable level of internal consistency. Higher scores on the index indicate greater support for the expansion of the state's economic role. Adhering to the sub-national perspective, the relationships of economic hardship and social capital with support for the expansion of the state's economic role were examined in the four regions of China, respectively. Figure 4.3 presents the results.

In the eastern region, no significant association was found between income decline and support for the expansion of the state's economic role. Social networks were negatively associated with support for the state's economic role ($b = -0.114$, $p = 0.035$), but social trust was positively associated with it ($b = 0.119$, $p = 0.019$). Additionally, older generations and highly educated people tended to support the expansion of the state's economic role ($b = 0.157$, $p = 0.003$; $b = 0.106$, $p = 0.041$).

In the central region, income decline was positively associated with support for the expansion of the state's economic role ($b = 0.198$, $p = 0.001$), while the three components of social capital were not. Regarding the demographic variables, males, highly educated people, and urban residents tended to support the expansion of the state's economic role ($b = -0.152$, $p = 0.027$; $b = 0.161$, $p = 0.032$; $b = 0.175$, $p = 0.019$).

In the western region, no significant association was found between income decline and support for the expansion of the state's economic role. Regarding

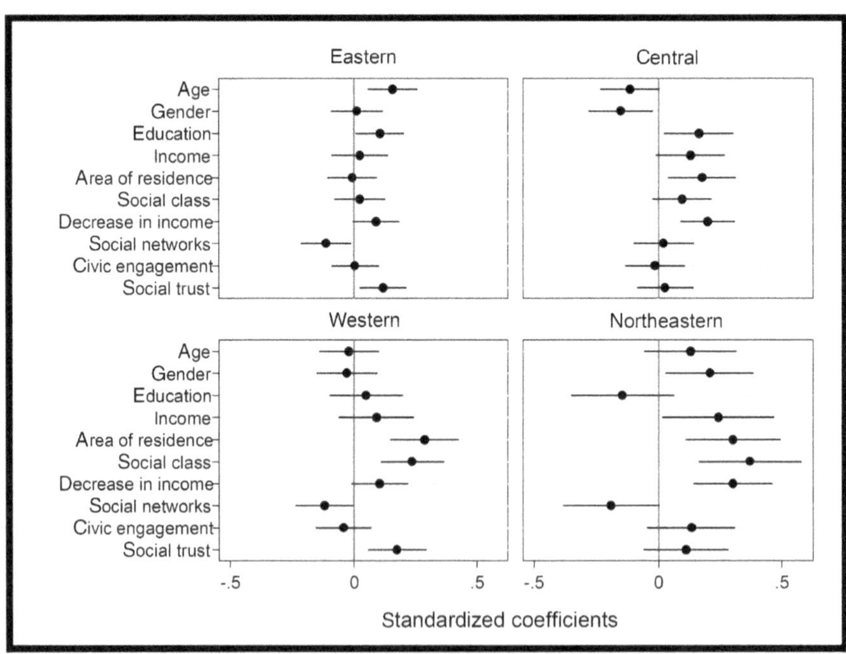

Figure 4.3 Predicting favorable attitudes toward the state's economic role.

social capital, social trust was positively associated with support for the expansion of the state's economic role ($b = 0.176$, $p = 0.006$). Regarding demographic attributes, urban residents and those with subjective membership to a high social class tended to support the expansion of the state's economic role ($b = 0.287$, $p < 0.001$; $b = 0.238$, $p = 0.001$).

In the northeastern region, income decline was positively associated with support for the expansion of the state's economic role ($b = 0.301$, $p = 0.002$), while the three components of social capital were not. Additionally, females, urban residents, and people with subjective membership to a high social class tended to support the expansion of the state's economic role ($b = 0.206$, $p = 0.042$; $b = 0.302$, $p = 0.007$; $b = 0.370$, $p = 0.003$).

Economic hardship in the eastern and western regions did not generate more support for the state's economic intervention among local citizens. The market-oriented economy is the strongest in the eastern region, where privately owned enterprises are active and create considerable wealth. Local people believe that the market-oriented economy is superior to the previously centralized planned economy. Even those whose income declined during the pandemic did not view the state's economic intervention as desirable. Given that the western region is situated in the national border area, far from the seat of central power, its residents may not have had a positive experience of the state's economic intervention. Therefore, when those individuals face economic hardship during the pandemic, they rarely consider the state's economic intervention as a preferable approach to improving their situation.

Regional variation also exists in the relationship between social capital and support for the expansion of the state's economic intervention. Since social capital can provide people with resources that may enable them to weather difficulties, the present study posited that people with considerable social capital might not support the state's economic intervention when they face economic hardship during the pandemic. The empirical results paint a complex picture. The three components of social capital had different effects on people's attitudes toward the state. Social networks indeed negatively predicted support for the state's economic intervention, but a significant association was only observed in the eastern region. Since the eastern region has the highest level of socioeconomic modernization, people with vast social networks can access more resources, and their efforts are rewarded in the market-oriented economy. Accordingly, such people did not view the expansion of the state's economic role as a favorable option, and they did not expect the state to intervene in economic activities. No significant relationship was found between civic engagement and attitude toward the state's economic intervention. Contrary to the prediction, social trust was positively associated with support for the state's economic intervention in the eastern and western regions. Previous studies found a positive relationship between social trust and support for the government (Bargsted et al., 2023; Dellmuth and Tallberg, 2020; Seifert, 2018). This chapter adds that this relationship holds in terms of support for the expansion of the state's economic role in China.

Conclusion

Since the initial COVID-19 outbreak in Wuhan in December 2019, China implemented the world's strictest countermeasures. Despite complaints about the inconvenience to ordinary life and loss of freedoms under the zero-COVID policy, the Chinese people showed a particularly high level of obedience to the authorities, and the state was able to enforce its stringent approach. To understand the dynamics of the citizen-state relationship, this chapter examined the Chinese citizenry's anti-COVID-19 policy preferences, their willingness to comply with the state's policy, and their support for expanding the state's economic intervention. It is worth noting that public opinion is volatile, and pandemic-related attitudes may have changed over time. As the data were collected in January 2022, the Omicron variant was not widely spread, and city-wide lockdowns were not prevalent. The results presented in this chapter primarily reflect the responses of the Chinese people to the pandemic during the first two years following the initial outbreak of COVID-19. However, long-lasting restrictions caused excessive harm to ordinary people, and the authorities underestimated the negative outcomes of the zero-COVID policy (Zeng, 2024; Zhai, 2023). Finally, by the end of 2022, widespread protests erupted, and this policy was terminated. Departing from the conventional approach that treats the country as a homogeneous object, the present study adopted a sub-national perspective and paid attention to regional differences. The survey data show that due to the pandemic, the proportion of people who have experienced income decline was relatively low in the eastern region but high in the northeastern region. Chinese people's willingness to comply with the state's anti-COVID-19 policy also varied by region. The results show that this analytical strategy is useful for identifying sub-national differences within China.

Value orientations affect Chinese citizens' COVID-19-related policy preferences. This chapter examined the influence of paternalist culture and liberal culture. Paternalist culture encourages individual dependence on the state, while liberal culture stresses individuals' autonomy and self-responsibility. Chinese citizens with paternalist values tended to perceive infection prevention and control as the state's responsibility, while those with liberal values believed that individuals should assume the brunt of the responsibility. The results show that attribution of responsibility to the state was positively associated with a preference for a policy that restricts freedom, whereas attribution of the responsibility for infection prevention and control to individuals was positively associated with a preference for a policy that prioritizes individual freedoms.

Policy preference and responsibility attribution influenced Chinese citizens' willingness to comply with the state's anti-COVID-19 policy. Preference for a policy that restricts freedom during the pandemic was positively associated with policy compliance. This finding was consistent in all four regions of China. The underlying logic is simple: People who supported the restriction of freedom were willing to comply with the zero-COVID policy, while those who prioritized individual freedoms resisted the policy. Moreover, the attribution of the responsibility for infection prevention and control to the state was positively associated with willingness to comply with the state's policy in the western and northeastern regions only. A similar relationship was not observed in the eastern and central regions. One possible explanation is the high level of economic modernization in the eastern and central regions and the limited influence of paternalist values there.

The zero-COVID policy has severely damaged China's economy. Many small and medium-sized businesses have been bankrupted, and people have lost their jobs. A crisis often provides an opportunity for the state to expand its power, as people have a higher tolerance for authoritarian power amid a crisis than they do in normal times. According to this logic, economic hardship during the pandemic might cause people to support the expansion of the state's economic role. However, factors that could balance the negative effects of economic hardship should also be considered. For example, social capital can provide people with the resources and support necessary to survive crises. Hence, this study scrutinized the effect of social capital on Chinese people's attitudes toward the state's economic role.

The results show regional variation in the effects of economic hardship and social capital on people's expectations of the state's economic role. Income decline motivated residents of the central and northeastern regions to support the expansion of the state's economic role, while a similar effect was not observed in the eastern and western regions. Regarding social capital, social networks negatively predicted support for the expansion of the state's economic role in the eastern region, but social trust positively predicted the same in the eastern and western regions. The results indicate heterogeneous characteristics for the three components of social capital. Social networks helped counterbalance the facilitating effect of economic hardship on people's support for the expansion of the state's economic role. People with larger social networks resisted the state's economic intervention. However, social trust had a positive association with support for the state's economic role. To some extent, social trust is connected to trust in political institutions. This positive relationship applies to the Chinese people's support for the state's economic role during the COVID-19 pandemic, as the crisis has given the state an opportunity to expand its power.

Chinese people's policy preferences, perceptions of the state's responsibility for infection prevention and control, willingness to comply with the state's anti-COVID-19 policy, and favorable attitudes toward the expansion of the state economic role all reflect the changing citizen-state relationship in China. The results of the analysis demonstrate the relevance of political culture to understanding the politics of the COVID-19 pandemic in China. The sub-national perspective is important for studying a diverse country such as China. Significant regional variation exists in Chinese people's attitudes toward state policy, affecting their policy compliance and expectations of the state. Chinese people's policy preferences, perceptions of the state's responsibility, policy compliance tendency, and expectations of the state in terms of economic intervention all provide a lens for understanding China's politics.

References

Almond, Gabriel and Sidney Verba. 1963. *The Civic Culture: Political Attitudes and Democracy in Five Nations*. Princeton, NJ: Princeton University Press.

Bargsted, Matías, Camila Ortiz, Ignacio Cáceres, and Nicolás M. Somma. 2023. Social and political trust in a low trust society. *Political Behavior* 45: 1401–1420.

Beugelsdijk, Sjoerd, Henri L. F. de Groot, and Anton B. T. M. van Schaik. 2004. Trust and economic growth: A robustness analysis. *Oxford Economic Papers* 56(1): 118–134.

Bjørnskov, Christian. 2012. How does social trust affect economic growth? *Southern Economic Journal* 78(4): 1346–1368.

Bourdieu, Pierre. 1986. The forms of capital. In John G Richardson (ed.), *Handbook of Theory and Research for the Sociology of Education*. New York: Greenwood Press, pp. 241–258.

Burt, Ronald S. 1992. *Structural Holes: The Social Structure of Competition*. Cambridge, MA: Harvard University Press.

Cattell, Vicky. 2001. Poor people, poor places, and poor health: The mediating role of social networks and social capital. *Social Science & Medicine* 52(10): 1501–1516.

Chen, Ji-Ming and Yi-Qing Chen. 2022. China can prepare to end its zero-COVID policy. *Nature Medicine* 28: 1104–1105.

Chu, Godwin and Yanan Yu. 1993. *The Great Wall in Ruins: Communication and Cultural Change in China*. Albany, NY: State University of New York Press.

Cook, Karen S. 2005. Networks, norms and trust: The social psychology of social capital. *Social Psychology Quarterly* 68(1): 4–14.

Crow, David, and Patti Waldmeir. 2020. US anti-lockdown protests: "If you are paranoid about getting sick, just don't go out." *Financial Times*, April 22, 2020. www.ft.com/content/15ca3a5f-bc5c-44a3-99a8-c446f6f6881c.

Dellmuth, Lisa Maria, and Jonas Tallberg. 2020. Why national and international legitimacy beliefs are linked: Social trust as an antecedent factor. *The Review of International Organizations* 15(2): 311–337.

Dickson, Bruce J., Mingming Shen, Jie Yan. 2017. Generating regime support in contemporary China: Legitimation and the local legitimacy deficit. *Modern China* 43(2): 123–155.

Fetzer, Joel S., and J. Christopher Soper. 2010. Confucian values and elite support for liberal democracy in Taiwan: The perils of priestly religion. *Politics and Religion* 3(3): 495–517.

Fukuyama, Francis. 2001. Social capital, civil society and development. *Third World Quarterly* 22(1): 7–20.

Gan, Nectar. 2022. "Voices of April": China's internet erupts in protest against censorship of Shanghai lockdown video. CNN, April 25, 2022. https://edition.cnn.com/2022/04/25/china/china-covid-beijing-shanghai-mic-intl-hnk/index.html.

Gan, Nectar and Shawn Deng. 2022. Chinese cities rush to lockdown in show of loyalty to Xi's "Zero-Covid" strategy. *CNN*, September 5. Accessed September 9, 2022, https://edition.cnn.com/2022/09/05/china/china-covid-lockdown-74-cities-intl-hnk/index.html.

Gan, Nectar and Selina Wang. 2022. At the heart of China's protests against Zero-Covid, young people cry for freedom. *CNN*, November 28. Accessed December 23, 2022, https://edition.cnn.com/2022/11/28/china/china-protests-covid-political-freedom-intl-hnk-mic/index.html.

Gao, Jingkang, and Jinhua Zhao. 2017. Normative and image motivations for transportation policy compliance. *Urban Studies* 54(14): 3318–3336.

Guan, Yue, Lei Guang, Lianjiang Li, and Yanchuan Liu. 2024. The rally effect of the COVID-19 pandemic and the White Paper Movement in China. *Journal of Contemporary China*, DOI: 10.1080/10670564.2024.2356863.

Hahm, Chaibong. 2004. The ironies of Confucianism. *Journal of Democracy* 15(3): 93–107.

Han, Guanghua and Yida Zhai. 2024a. Temporary food insecurity, social capital, and mental health during the COVID-19 lockdowns in Shanghai. *Journal of Urban Affairs*, DOI: 10.1080/07352166.2024.2393840.

Han, Guanghua and Yida Zhai. 2024b. The association between food insecurity and social capital under the lockdowns in COVID-hit Shanghai. *Urban Studies* 61(1): 130–147.

Hogg, Michael A. 2005. Social identity and misuse of power: The dark side of leadership. *Brooklyn Law Review* 70(4): 1239–1257.

Hogg, Michael A. 2007. Organizational orthodoxy and corporate autocrats: Some nasty consequences of organizational identification in uncertain times. In Caroline A. Bartel, Steven Blader, and Amy Wrzesniewski (eds.), *Identity and the Modern Organization*. Mahwah, NJ: Erlbaum, pp. 35–59.

Hua, Shiping. 2001. *Chinese Political Culture 1989-2000*. Armonk, NY: M. E. Sharpe.

Iddiols, Rob and Jo Shelley. 2021. Violent clashes erupt during anti-lockdown demonstrations in Europe. *CNN*, November 22, 2021. https://edition.cnn.com/2021/11/21/europe/europe-lockdown-protests-violence-intl/index.html

Inglehart, Ronald, and Christian Welzel. 2005. *Modernization, Cultural Change, and Democracy: The Human Development Sequence*. Cambridge: Cambridge University Press.

Keng, Shu, Lingna Zhong, and Fang Xie. 2024. Why did China's zero-COVID policy persist? Decision urgency, regime type, and political opportunity structures. *Journal of Contemporary China* 33(146): 206–222.

Knack, Stephen and Philip Keefer. 1997. Does social capital have an economic payoff? A cross-country investigation. *Quarterly Journal of Economics* 62(4): 1251–1288.

Kornai, János. 1980. *Economics of Shortage*. Amsterdam: North-Holland Publishing Co.

Lei, Ya-Wen. 2020. Revisiting China's social volcano: Attitudes toward inequality and political trust in China. *Socius: Sociological Research for a Dynamic World* 6: 1–21.

Lewis-Beck, Michael S., Wenfang Tang, and Nicholas F. Martini. 2014. A Chinese popularity function sources of government support. *Political Research Quarterly* 67(1): 16–25.

Li, Bin, Tuo Li, Man Yu, and Bin Chen. 2017. Can equalization of public services narrow the regional disparities in China? A spatial econometrics approach. *China Economic Review* 44: 67–78.

Lin, Nan. 2001. *Social Capital: A Theory of Social Structure and Action*. Cambridge: Cambridge University Press.

Liu, Kerry. 2021. COVID-19 and the Chinese economy: Impacts, policy responses and implications. *International Review of Applied Economics* 35(2): 308–330.

Liu, Shu-hsien. 1996. Confucian ideals and the real world. In Wei-ming Tu (ed.), *Confucian Traditions in East Asian Modernity*. Cambridge, MA: Harvard University Press, pp. 92–112.

Mandarano, Lynn, Mahbubur Meenar, and Christopher Steins. 2010. Building social capital in the digital age of civic engagement. *Journal of Planning Literature* 25(2): 123–135.

Martín, Ana M., Bernardo Hernández, Martha Frías-Armenta, Stephany Hess. 2012. Why ordinary people comply with environmental laws: A structural model on normative and attitudinal determinants of illegal anti-ecological behaviour. *Legal and Criminological Psychology* 19(1): 80–103.

Nahapiet, Janine and Sumantra Ghoshal. 1998. Social capital, intellectual capital, and the organizational advantage. *Academy of Management Review* 23(2): 242–266.

Norris, Pippa. 2002. *Democratic Phoenix: Reinventing Political Activism*. Cambridge: Cambridge University Press.

Putnam, Robert D. 1993. *Making Democracy Work: Civic Traditions in Modern Italy*. Princeton, NJ: Princeton University Press.

Putnam, Robert D. 1995. Bowling alone: America's declining social capital. *Journal of Democracy* 6(1): 65–78.

Sanyal, Saswata, and Jayant K. Routray. 2016. Social capital for disaster risk reduction and management with empirical evidences from Sundarbans of India. *International Journal of Disaster Risk Reduction* 19: 101–111.

Seifert, Nico. 2018. Yet another case of Nordic exceptionalism? Extending existing evidence for a causal relationship between institutional and social trust to the Netherlands and Switzerland. *Social Indicators Research* 136(2): 539–555.

Shen, Zhongwen. 2022. The dynamic zero-COVID approach is the only way to defeat the virus. *Shenzhen Special Zone Daily*, March 20, 2022. http://sztqb.sznews.com/MB/content/202203/20/content_1177355.html.

Shi, Tianjian. 2014. *The Cultural Logic of Politics in Mainland China and Taiwan*. Cambridge: Cambridge University Press.

Subramanian, S. V., Ichiro Kawachi, and Bruce Kennedy. 2001. Does the state you live in make a difference? Multilevel analysis of self-rated health in the US. *Social Science & Medicine* 53(1): 9–19.

Talhelm, Thomas, Xuemin Zhang, Shigehiro Oishi, C. Shimin, D. Duan, X. Lan, and Shinobu Kitayama. 2014. Large-scale psychological differences within China explained by rice versus wheat agriculture. *Science* 344(6184): 603–608.

Welzel, Christian, Ronald Inglehart, and Franziska Deutsch. 2005. Social capital, voluntary associations and collective action: Which aspects of social capital have the greatest "civic" payoff? *Journal of Civil Society* 1(2): 121–146.

Whiteley, Paul. 2000. Economic growth and social capital. *Political Studies* 48(3): 443–466.

Woods, Eric Taylor, Robert Schertzer, Liah Greenfeld, Chris Hughes, and Cynthia Miller-Idriss. 2020. COVID-19, nationalism, and the politics of crisis: A scholarly exchange. *Nations and Nationalism* 26(4): 807–825.

Wright, Arthur F. 1975. *Confucianism and Chinese Civilization*. Stanford, CA: Stanford University Press.

Wu, Cary, Zhilei Shi, Rima Wilkes, Jiaji Wu, Zhiwen Gong, et al. 2021. Chinese citizen satisfaction with government performance during COVID-19. *Journal of Contemporary China* 30(132): 930–944.

Xi Jinping. 2020. Remarks at the meeting to commend role models in the country's fight against the COVID-19 epidemic. September 8, 2020. www.gov.cn/xinwen/2020-10/15/content_5551552.htm

Xie, Yu, and Xiang Zhou. 2014. Income inequality in today's China. *Proceedings of the National Academy of Sciences of the United States of America* 111(19): 6928–6933.

Xinhua News Agency. 2022. The Standing Committee of the Political Bureau of the CCP Central Committee had a meeting to analyze the current epidemic prevention and control situation, discuss priorities, and make arrangements for relevant work. May 5, 2022. www.ccdi.gov.cn/toutiaon/202205/t20220505_190694_m.html.

Yagil, Dana. 1998. Instrumental and normative motives for compliance with traffic laws among young and older drivers. *Accident Analysis & Prevention* 30(4): 417–424.

Yao, Xinzhong. 2000. *An Introduction to Confucianism*. Cambridge: Cambridge University Press.

Zeng, Qingjie. 2024. Strict COVID-19 lockdown and popular regime support in China. *Democratization* 31(7): 1373–1396.

Zhai, Yida. 2017. Values of deference to authority in Japan and China. *International Journal of Comparative Sociology* 58(2): 120–139.

Zhai, Yida. 2021. Sources of political trust and their regional variations in China. *Social Science Journal*, DOI:10.1080/03623319.2021.1922976.

Zhai, Yida. 2022. Values change and support for democracy in East Asia. *Social Indicators Research* 160(1): 179–198.

Zhai, Yida. 2023. The politics of COVID-19: The political logic of China's Zero-COVID policy. *Journal of Contemporary Asia* 53(5): 869–886.

Zhai, Yida. 2024. Outgroup threat, ideology, and favorable evaluations of the government's responses to COVID-19. *Current Psychology* 43: 13110–13119.

Zhai, Yida and Guanghua Han. 2024. Lockdown, information quality, and political trust: An empirical study of the Shanghai lockdown under COVID-19. *International Review of Administrative Sciences* 90(1): 132–148.

Zhang, Xinxin, Wenhong Zhang, and Saijuan Chen. 2022. Shanghai's life-saving efforts against the current omicron wave of the COVID-19 pandemic. *The Lancet* 399(10340): 2011–2012.

Zhao, Yu, Hongyuan Zhang, Yibing Ding, and Sitong Tang. 2021. Implications of COVID-19 pandemic on China's exports. *Emerging Markets Finance and Trade* 57(6): 1716–1726.

Zhou, Yingnan Joseph and Shuai Jin. 2018. Inequality and political trust in China: The social volcano thesis reexamined. *China Quarterly* 236: 1033–1062.

Part II

Comparative Perspectives on State-Society Relations in East Asia

5 Asian Values and Restrictions on Freedom

Hidehiro Yamamoto

Introduction

During the COVID-19 pandemic, the relationship between the state and society faced great challenges, especially in liberal democratic regimes. Restraining the spread of the pandemic required the controlling of human behavior as well as medical countermeasures. The measures included mandatory mask-wearing, restrictions on movement between areas, bans on gatherings and events, and limitations on the operations of restaurants and other businesses. In some countries, legal measures such as lockdowns were employed, significantly restricting the overall life of citizens. Additionally, certain governments utilized digital technology to monitor the behavior of their citizens.

The implementation of these measures typically involved the exercise of authority over citizens, which is often viewed as an undesirable aspect of a liberal democratic regime. The suppression of contagious diseases is a collective duty that necessitates the cooperation of individual initiatives (Cato et al., 2020). As per Thomas Hobbes' philosophical principles, state-imposed measures are the most effective means of achieving this objective.[1] During the COVID-19 pandemic, restrictions on individual freedoms were deemed necessary by even liberal democratic regimes as well as authoritarian governments.[2] However, coercion by the state does not necessarily bring about the internalization of behavioral change in people. This is where the functioning of shared norms within society is indispensable (Marti'nez, 2021; Neville et al., 2021). Neville et al. (2021) insisted on the importance of social identity as a member of a group.

Conversely, the behavioral limitations imposed by the COVID-19 pandemic have had a profound impact on the economy. Specifically, limitations on dining out, travel or sightseeing, or public events have resulted in a loss of income for those in related industries. If citizens' economic activities were harmed by state control, the responsibility of the state to provide compensation was considered. Therefore, many governments provided financial assistance to compensate for the enforced time off work. Other economic stimulus measures were also adopted to restore the overall cooling of economic activity.

DOI: 10.4324/9781003495239-7

However, such state coercion and compensation conflicted with the trend toward economic liberalism. In capitalist regimes, the stalemate of the welfare state since the 1970s has led to calls for more market-based principles, less state intervention, individual autonomy, and self-responsibility (Harvey, 2005; Steger and Roy, 2010).

In contrast, the economic policy implemented in response to COVID-19 was characterized by significant state intervention and social democratic principles. Given the dire financial situation faced by each country, the increase in spending was a subject of much debate and controversy. Actually, in the United States, the ideological conflict between conservatives and liberals over COVID-19 measures had arisen (Gollwitzer, 2020; Kerr et al., 2021).

It is essential to consider how citizens evaluated the advisability of state intervention during the COVID-19 pandemic, given the restrictions on freedom and the financial support provided. Public support for government policies is crucial in democratic regimes. Furthermore, the active participation of citizens is crucial for the successful execution of policies, including in non-democratic systems, and this was even more so during the COVID-19 pandemic when the extent of state intervention was significantly greater.

COVID-19 Policy Support and Asian Values

To what extent did citizens in Japan, Korea, and China support the government's COVID-19 measures? What may have prompted this support? The primary objective of the current chapter is a comparative examination of the degree to which the general public has endorsed state initiatives aimed at curbing the propagation of COVID-19 in Japan, Korea, and China.

These countries in East Asia have achieved noteworthy success in preventing the spread of COVID-19 infections. This observation has generated interest in the possibility of a distinct factor that may be present in East Asia. Shinya Yamanaka, who won the Nobel Prize in Physiology or Medicine, termed this "Factor X." One of the objectives of this chapter is to explore Factor X from a sociopolitical viewpoint.

Japan and Korea are both liberal democracies, while China is a one-party ruling system. The disparities in political systems can be seen as national ideals. In liberal democratic countries, individual freedom and privacy are considered fundamental human rights that must be respected, whereas, in authoritarian regimes, these rights are not always upheld. Instead, such regimes tend to tolerate violations of freedom and privacy as a result of their submissive attitude toward a strong state or leader.

Although democracies prioritize individual rights, these rights may be temporarily suspended during emergencies to protect public welfare. In certain countries, the implementation of COVID-19 measures has led to lockdowns that significantly restrict citizens' lives. Emergencies often elicit a "rally around the flag" effect, which can increase citizens' support for their governments (Baekgaard et al., 2020; Dominik, 2021; Hegewald and Schraff, 2024).

It is often posited that a shared cultural heritage is prevalent in East Asian countries, despite their disparate political systems. In the Inglehart-Welzel Cultural

Map based on the World Values Survey, these three countries are included in the Confucian culture cluster (World Value Survey website[3]). The cultural practices that are distinct from those of the West are deeply ingrained in Confucianism and characterized by Asian values (Fukuyama, 1995; Zakaria and Yew, 1994). Asian values were once a controversial issue in the 1990s with the rise of Korea and Southeast Asian countries. That is, East Asia successfully developed economies based on values different from Western-style liberal democracy.

Although the values held by Asians are multifaceted, Kim (2010) specifically identified four dimensions for empirical examination. One of these dimensions is familism, which underscores the importance of respecting and obeying one's parents, not only in private but also in public settings. The second is communalism, in which the group is prioritized over individual welfare and freedom. The third is authoritarianism, which includes obedience to those in authority or power and governing by consensus rather than competition. The fourth is ethics in work and education.

There are many other arguments for Asian values. What many of these discussions have in common is that Asian values emphasize vertical relationships and a harmonious orientation (Dalton and Shin, 2006; Ikeda, 2021). They also place emphasis on respect for superiors and those in authority, as well as the need to prioritize the collective good over individual interests. Instead, those in positions of authority have a responsibility to safeguard their subordinates. These relationships extend to the political realm, as well as social or private spheres. This perspective encompasses paternalism and authoritarianism, where the state is viewed as a parent, prioritizing national interest and preserving social order.

However, the values prevalent in Asia are not compatible with the principles of liberal democracy, which emphasizes individual freedom and rights. This discord has been a prominent theme. Several empirical investigations have been carried out in various Asian nations (Dalton and Shin, 2006; Dalton and Ong, 2005; Kim, 2010; Park and Shin, 2006; Zhai, 2016), yet the outcomes have been inconclusive.

Nevertheless, if individuals possess Asian values, they could encourage cooperation and support for measures implemented by the government in response to COVID-19. This is because the hierarchical relationship and group priority of Asian values are the norms that make the group follow their rules.

However, the influence of values may vary based on the political system. Since both Japan and Korea are liberal democracies, even if they hold Asian values, there may be conflicting values present. Conversely, in China, an authoritarian regime, Asian values may have a more significant impact.

This chapter aims to examine, through a comparative analysis of the three countries, whether political systems and cultural values influence attitudes toward the policy. Through a questionnaire survey, we collect data on the level of support among citizens in each country for Asian values, restrictions on freedom for the purpose of curbing the spread of COVID-19, and measures to mitigate the economic impact caused by the pandemic. We then investigate the correlation between Asian values and policy support, as well as the variations among the countries.

Analysis

Authoritarian Attitudes as Asian Values

(1) Distribution of Asian Values

According to the survey data, we initially assess the distribution of Asian values in each country. We define Asian values as vertical relationships and harmony within the group, utilizing the following four questions.

Vertical relationships:
- We must always pay respect to those in authority.
- In times of emergency, it is better to obey government requests to restrict freedom of speech.
- We need strong leadership to overcome social difficulties.

Group harmony:
- People should be prepared to sacrifice their personal interests for the sake of the nation and society.
- If people's ideas are too diverse, society becomes disorderly.

These questions were rated on a 7-point scale, with higher scores signifying a more positive outlook. This means that the Asian value is higher. The mean values for each country are illustrated in Figure 5.1. Generally, the mean score in China was quite high. Specifically, for vertical relationships, respect for authority figures, and restrictions on freedom of speech during emergencies, the scores were particularly high. In contrast, Japan and Korea had mean scores of around 4.0, which is in the middle of the scale. All three countries had positive views on strong leadership, with mean scores above 5.0.

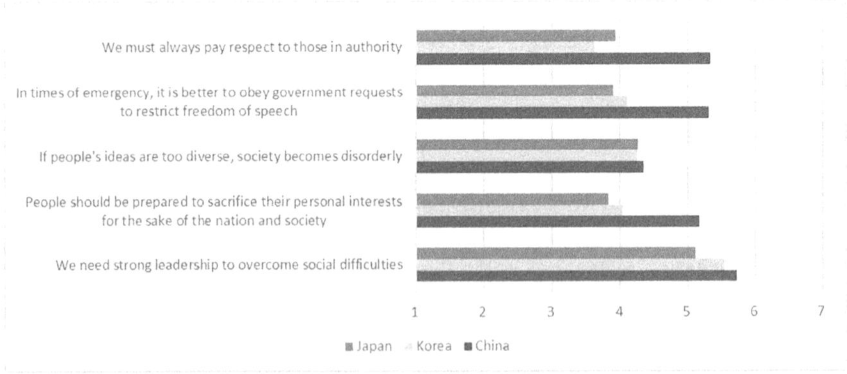

Figure 5.1 Support for Asian values: Mean on 7-point scale.

When it came to group harmony, there was little difference among the three countries in terms of diverse opinions and disorder. However, the mean value for self-sacrifice for the nation and society was higher in China.

These findings suggest that China supports Asian values related to social hierarchy and group primacy. The other two countries did not have negative attitudes toward these anti-liberal democratic values, but there was no clear pattern.

(2) Asian Values and Education and Generation

However, authoritarian attitudes are likely to vary according to education. That is, the higher the level of education, the more liberal the values one acquires (Schuman et al., 1992; Stubager, 2008). The three Asian countries are now known as societies that place importance on educational attainment.

With industrialization, academic credentials became highly prized, and competition for entrance examinations intensified. Consequently, it is reasonable to expect that the younger generation will be more highly educated and will exhibit a greater distance from Asian values. Furthermore, different generations within the three countries have experienced distinct political and social dynamics as they navigate significant social transformations. Therefore, the effect of both cohort and education should be examined.

Table 5.1 presents the mean of Asian values for each country, categorized by educational attainment and birth cohort. Education level was considered high if the respondent held a university degree or graduate school diploma, and low if they did not attend university. The birth cohort was divided into ten-year intervals, ranging from the 1950s to the 1990s. Given the strong correlation among the aforementioned five items (Cronbach's $\alpha = 0.780$), they were explicitly summed and combined into a single-dimensional measure for Asian values. The minimum value of the scale was 5.0, the maximum value was 35.0, the mean was 22.8, and the standard deviation was 5.8.

Table 5.1 Mean of Asian values of each country by birth cohort and education

Birth cohorts	*Japan*		*Korea*		*China*	
	high education	*Low education*	*high education*	*Low education*	*high education*	*Low education*
1950s	19.6	21.1	22.2	24.0	-	21.1
1960s	20.3	20.9	21.3	22.8	32.0	25.4
1970s	20.3	21.3	20.7	21.2	25.8	27.6
1980s	20.9	22.4	20.9	21.0	25.3	27.1
1990s	22.1	22.3	20.8	23.2	26.0	25.7
Total	20.6	21.5	21.1	22.6	25.8	25.9

Japan exhibited a relatively low overall level of Asian values. However, generational differences were also slight but tended to be higher among the younger generations. It is worth mentioning that the authoritarian attitudes prevalent among the younger respondents aligned with the findings of other social surveys conducted in Japan (Kikkawa, 2014, chapter 6; Matsutani, 2014). Although the difference was not substantial, individuals with higher levels of education tended to possess lower Asian values.

Koreans from the 1950s-born cohort tended to support Asian values, although this sentiment declined and leveled off among the more educated younger generations. Among the less-educated, support for Asian values continued to decline within the younger generation after those born in the 1960s (the so-called 386 generation), who led the democracy movement in the 1980s. However, such support was growing among the less-educated born in the 1990s.

The data indicates that China demonstrated higher levels of internalization of Asian values compared to the other two countries. For individuals with lower levels of education, this degree of internalization was not significant for those born in the 1950s, but it increased over subsequent generations and decreased for those born in the 1990s. Among the highly educated, those born in the 1950s were not included in the sample, and the results for those born in the 1960s were limited due to the small sample size of eight. However, for those born in the 1970s and beyond, the mean score was slightly lower than that of the less-educated and those further from the values of Asian culture.

The extent of support for Asian values varied across countries and was influenced by the level of education. Less-educated individuals in each country tended to hold more Asian values, while the degree of support for these values differed among different cohorts.

Role of the State in COVID-19 Measures

Let us now investigate the attitudes toward COVID-19 measures. Initially, we assessed citizens' understanding of the government's role in each country. Figure 5.2 presents the mean of a 7-point scale question soliciting opinions on the overall policy. Is the prevention of COVID-19 a public good that should be addressed by the state, or is it an individual responsibility? When the survey inquired as to whether preventing infection or recovering from the economic blow (with economic recovery scoring higher) was more crucial, the mean value for both was above the median value of 4.0, implying that citizens in each country generally placed greater importance on preventing infection. This is especially evident in China, where the mean value is as high as 5.4 (Japan 4.8, South Korea 4.6).

All three countries expressed a favorable view on the notion that "To prevent infection, it is inevitable that personal freedom is restricted," with high mean values recorded in China (5.2), followed by Japan (4.9) and Korea (4.6). Additionally, China showed a high mean value of 5.5 for the statement "We should fully comply with the government's corona measures, no matter how inconvenient they may

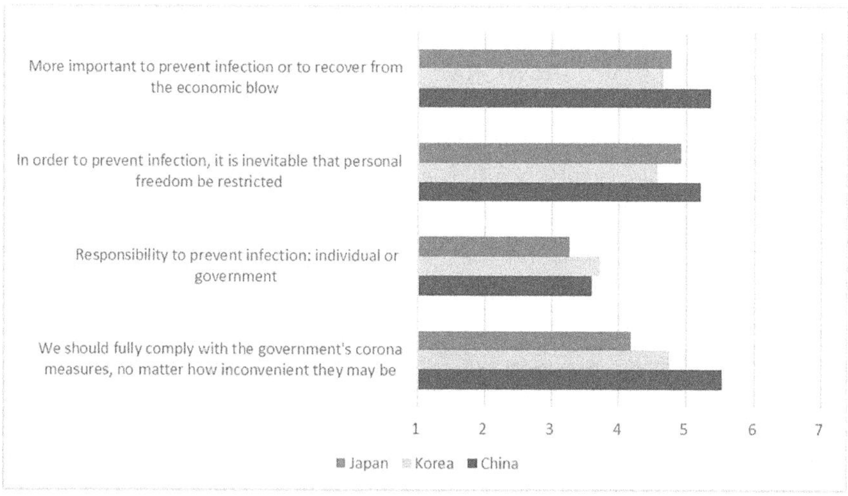

Figure 5.2 Role of the state in COVID-19 measures (mean of 7-point scales).

be," with Korea (4.7) and Japan (4.2) recording lower but still significant mean values.

Lastly, after evaluating the role of individuals and governments in preventing infection, the survey participants were found to be more inclined toward the responsibility of individuals, compared to an intermediate level of responsibility assigned to the government, in all three countries. The mean score for Japan was 3.3, which was lower than the scores of 3.7 and 3.6, respectively, for Korea and China. This suggests a relatively stronger inclination toward considering individuals as primarily responsible for preventing infections.

The three countries have placed a strong emphasis on the prevention of infection at the start of 2022 and are willing to accept limitations on their freedoms imposed by the state. This approach aligns with Asian values, and such an attitude is particularly evident in China, a country with a one-party-dominant political system that has pursued a zero-coronavirus policy. In contrast, Japan tends to accept more restrictions on freedom, but the population often disregards the government's guidelines and views infection prevention as a personal responsibility. This can be seen as a preference for community-based prevention measures rather than state-imposed restrictions.

Evaluation of Individual COVID-19 Measures

The analysis subsequently focused on assessing the effectiveness of COVID-19 measures that entailed limitations on individual freedom or mandatory actions (illustrated in Figure 5.3). The graph depicts the mean of countries for post-vaccination restrictions concerning food and drink consumption, travel, digital

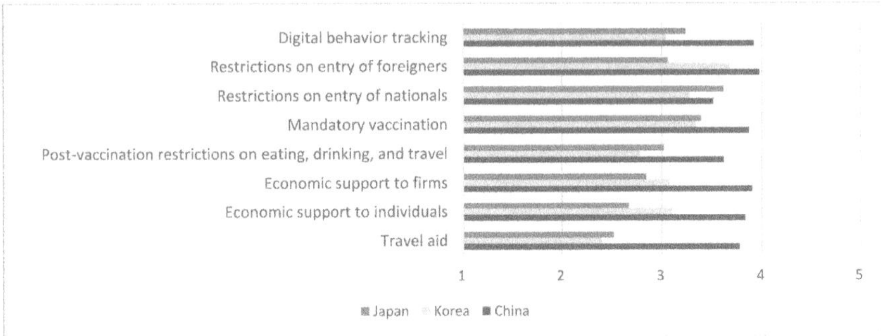

Figure 5.3 Evaluation of COVID-19 measures and financial aids (mean on a 5-point scale).

behavior tracking, restrictions on foreigners' entry, restrictions on nationals' entry, and mandatory vaccination. Each of the aforementioned measures was evaluated on a 5-point scale.

China's mean for these items demonstrated strong support for the government's COVID-19 measures, with values ranging from 3.5 to 4.0. Notably high scores were observed for the restrictions on foreigners entering the country (4.0), digital behavior tracking (3.9), and mandatory vaccination (3.9).

In contrast, the support levels demonstrated by Japan and Korea were not so high, although their mean were typically greater than 3.0. Even so, Japan and Korea exhibited relatively high scores for entry restrictions for foreigners, with values of 3.6 and 3.7, respectively, for foreigners, and 3.4 and 3.3, respectively, for domestic cases. These differences from those observed in China were relatively small, which may indicate caution against the spread of the infection through overseas travel.

However, the scores for digital activity tracking were significantly different, with values of 3.1 and 3.0 in Japan and Korea, respectively, compared to 3.9 in China. This large difference in the advanced surveillance technology of digital tracking can be seen as an indication of differences in attitudes toward human rights. Authoritarian regimes emphasized the deterrence of overall infection rather than individual privacy. It is interesting to note that the evaluation of citizens in Korea, where digital tracking was actually introduced, and in Japan, where it was not, remained almost the same.

The differences between Japan and Korea suggest that Korea was more supportive of mandatory vaccination (Korea 3.3 vs. Japan 3.0), while Japan was more supportive of restrictions on post-vaccination behavior (Japan 3.2 vs. Korea 2.8). It can be assumed that Korea has a higher evaluation of vaccine effectiveness as a preventive measure.

The bottom three policies in Figure 5.3 illustrate the assessment of three economic support measures: support to individuals and families, support to firms, and travel aid. Just as with behavioral restrictions, China's mean of 3.8–3.9 was higher than that of the other two countries. In response to economic damage, Korea scored higher than Japan in providing aid to firms and individuals/families, with a score of 3.1. However, there was no significant difference between Japan and Korea in terms of travel subsidies, which is a more aggressive economic stimulus measure.

Asian Values and Policy Evaluation

Turning our focus toward the influence of Asian values on the assessment of COVID-19 policies in each country, it is considered that individuals who exhibit increased obedience to government authorities and demonstrate a preference for social harmony are more likely to endorse the restrictive measures put in place in response to the pandemic. Furthermore, economic support from the government is also anticipated to be shaped by Asian values. Specifically, the greater people value vertical relationships and social harmony, the higher the esteem in which the government's actions will be held.

This study aims to evaluate the impact of Asian values across three countries. As previously stated, we expect the influence of these values to be most pronounced in China, a nation with an authoritarian political system. So far, China has recorded the highest scores in both Asian values and support for COVID-19 measures. To investigate this issue, multiple regression analyses was conducted, considering the relevant variables.

Specifically, an additive scale of the five variables previously mentioned (namely respect for people in authority, limited freedom of speech in times of emergency, desire for strong leadership, dedication to the state and society, and disorderly social diversity) was utilized for Asian values. Dummy variables for Korea and China were entered, with Japan serving as the reference category. Furthermore, I assessed the variations in the relationship between Asian values and policy evaluation across countries by introducing an interaction term between each country and the Asian value scale. In authoritarian China, the influence of Asian values is more pronounced, while in liberal democratic Japan and Korea, the effect may be more restricted.

Previous analysis revealed that Asian values differ based on birth cohort and educational level in each country. As such, we controlled these factors by utilizing the cohort (born in the 50s, 60s, 70s, 80s, and 90s) and education level (university graduate or higher or less than university graduate) as variables. Sex was also considered.

The findings from the multiple regression analysis with COVID-19 measures and behavioral restrictions as dependent variables are presented in Table 5.2. By concentrating on Asian values, I scrutinized these results.

Digital tracking, restrictions on citizen and foreigner entry, and mandatory vaccinations yielded largely similar outcomes. The impact of Asian values was generally positive and statistically significant. Its interaction effect with Korea

Table 5.2 Impact of Asian values on the evaluation of COVID-19 measures: multiple regression analyses

		Post-vaccination Restrictions on events		*Digital tracking*		*Restrictions on the entry of domestic nationals*		*Restrictions on the entry of foreigners*		*Vaccine mandates*	
		b	*S.E.*	*b*	*S.E.*	*B*	*S.E.*	*b*	*S.E.*	*b*	*S.E.*
Country	Korea	−0.573	0.192**	−0.391	0.173*	0.023	0.186	−0.201	0.187	0.308	0.194
	China	0.147	0.229	0.114	0.207	−0.446	0.222*	−0.772	0.223**	0.393	0.231
	Ref: Japan										
Asian value		−0.015	0.007*	0.046	0.006**	0.041	0.006**	0.038	0.006**	0.061	0.007**
	Korea × Asian value	0.007	0.009	0.015	0.008	0.000	0.008	0.002	0.008	0.000	0.009
	China × Asian value	0.015	0.009	0.021	0.008*	0.023	0.009*	0.026	0.009**	0.012	0.010
Cohorts	50s	0.265	0.067**	0.086	0.060	−0.003	0.065	−0.187	0.066**	0.491	0.068**
	60s	0.182	0.060**	0.057	0.054	−0.014	0.580	−0.072	0.058	0.323	0.060**
	70s	0.114	0.062	0.070	0.055	0.009	0.060	0.025	0.060	0.171	0.062*
	80s	−0.004	0.058	0.003	0.053	0.115	0.056*	0.092	0.057	0.100	0.059
	Ref: 90s										
Sex	Male	−0.082	0.039*	0.084	0.035*	-0.095	0.038*	−0.056	0.038	0.098	0.040*
Education	University graduate	−0.013	0.410	0.146	0.037**	0.024	0.040	−0.044	0.040	0.064	0.042
Constant		3.488	0.009**	1.931	0.139**	2.772	0.149**	2.678	0.150**	1.419	0.156**
Adjusted R^2		0.101		0.225		0.082		0.070		0.184	
N		3000		3000		3000		3000		3000	

* $p < .05$, ** $p < .01$ (** p<.01).

was insignificant for all measures. In contrast, the interaction term between Asian values and China was positively statistical significant, with the exception of the vaccine mandate. That is, the slope of Asian value for China was particularly steep, indicating that the authoritarian regime enhanced the effectiveness of Asian values.

Asian values exhibited a negative and statistically significant influence on post-vaccination constraints related to eating, drinking, and travel. No interaction effects were apparent for any country. In simple terms, individuals with higher levels of Asian values tended to rate behavioral restrictions more negatively, regardless of the country they resided in. This finding contrasts with the expectations outlined in the current chapter. One reason for this may be that we asked about the situation after vaccination. In other words, people with Asian values may have expressed support for the premise that they followed the government's instructions in vaccinating and rather tolerated the freedom of action that followed.

In addition, the main effect of Korea is smaller than that of Japan. This is confirmed by the earlier comparison of means among countries, but it can be stated that Korea has a higher evaluation of the effectiveness of the vaccine as a preventive measure.

The consequences of sociodemographic variables varied depending on the measures. For the birth cohort, post-vaccination restrictions and vaccine mandates showed a favorable statistical correlation for those born in the 50s and 60s as compared to those born in the 90s. The elderly were more prudent. With regard to the entry restrictions for domestic nationals, those born in the 80s experienced a favorable effect when compared to those born in the 90s. No cohort effects were observed for digital tracking or entry restrictions for foreign nationals.

Sex did not exhibit a consistent pattern across measures. Digital tracking and vaccine mandates showed a positive correlation and received greater support from males. In contrast, post-vaccination restrictions and entry restrictions for domestic nationals demonstrated a negative correlation and received greater support from women. No gender effect was detected for entry restrictions for foreign nationals. Higher education was more supportive of digital tracking, but no effect was observed for the other measures.

Table 5.3 shows the outcomes of the multiple regression analysis, with the economic support policy serving as the dependent variable. As per the findings, it was discovered that Asian values had a positive impact on both of these policies. Moreover, a favorable interaction effect between Asian values and China was observed for economic support provided to firms and individuals. This mirrors the stronger effect of Asian values in China. Regarding travel aid, no significant interaction effect was observed; however, the effect was more pronounced in China compared to Japan.

Table 5.3 Impact of Asian values on the evaluation of economic support: multiple regression analyses

		Economic support to firms		*Economic support to individuals*		*Travel aid*	
	Asian value	0.041	0.006**	0.043	0.006**	0.050	0.006**
Country	Korea	0.224	0.166	0.642	0.183**	−0.008	0.176
	China	0.075	0.198	−0.170	0.218	0.590	0.210**
	Ref: Japan						
	Korea × Asian Value	0.000	0.008	−0.010	0.008	−0.007	0.008
	China × Asian Value	0.031	0.008**	0.045	0.009**	0.014	0.009
Cohorts	50s	0.106	0.058	0.120	0.064	−0.252	0.061**
	60s	−0.008	0.052	−0.021	0.057	−0.208	0.055**
	70s	−0.035	0.053	−0.044	0.058	−0.102	0.056
	80s	0.014	0.050	−0.042	0.055	−0.071	0.053
	Ref: 90s						
Sex	Male	0.009	0.034	−0.065	0.037	0.036	0.036
education	university graduate	0.059	0.036	−0.010	0.039	0.014	0.038
Constant		1.929	0.133	1.787	0.147**		
Adjusted R^2		0.249		0.24		0.331	
N		3000		3000		3000	

* (* p<.05) $p < .05$, ** $p < .01$.

Conclusion

This chapter offers a comparative examination of the assessments made by citizens regarding the measures undertaken in response to COVID-19 in Japan, Korea, and China, with a particular emphasis on the expression of Asian values related to vertical relationship and group harmony. The following is a concise summary of the results obtained:

Initially, all three countries prioritized the prevention of infection over economic recovery during the sixth wave of the pandemic. This led them to accept state intervention that restricted their freedom. It is evident that the positive perception of the state's role in COVID-19 control extended beyond the differences in the political systems of East Asian countries. Additionally, with the exception of post-vaccination restrictions on eating, drinking, and travel, many COVID-19 measures were widely supported, as they aligned with Asian values. Consequently, it can be inferred that the level of support for COVID-19 measures in each country depends on the extent to which Asian values are internalized.

These trends were particularly evident in China, where citizens had a strong sense of Asian values and were generally accepting of restrictions on their freedom to curb the spread of infection. Additionally, support for measures to combat COVID-19 was closely linked to the prevalence of Asian values. Although the influence of these values was present in all countries, in China, with its one-party-dominant political system, state authority served as the foundation for policy support.

Generally, there were no substantial discernible differences between Japan and Korea. Although Asian values played a role, there was no observable interaction effect between Japanese and Korean values, and the impacts are roughly comparable. Due to their democratic systems, they did not display the same robust authoritarian inclinations as China; however, their underlying cultural values seemed to be present.

It appears that the social hierarchies and group primacy that are prevalent in East Asian societies have contributed to the acceptance of state intervention in the region, which can be seen in the success of COVID-19 measures, also known as Factor X. However, these values conflict with the principles of liberal democracy, which prioritize individual freedom and rights. This is despite the presence of democratic systems in countries such as Japan and Korea. There is a paradoxical aspect to this situation, as popular support for policies is based on values that deviate from those of liberal democracies.

However, it is possible that this is not solely due to Asian values. In recent years, there have been populist arguments in democratic politics that combine distrust of the political establishment with a desire for stronger leaders who represent the voices of radical citizens (Hawkins et al., 2017; Mudde and Kaltwasser, 2017). If this is the case, there may be support for policy implementation under strong leaders, not just in East Asian countries. It is important to note that this should not be taken as a criticism of East Asian societies, but rather an observation of the complexities of democratic politics.

Certainly, further exploration of other East Asian regions and comparison with other regions, including the West, are necessary to confirm this. Additionally, the examination of supportive attitudes toward policies other than COVID-19 countermeasures would provide valuable insights. However, the discussion in this chapter has successfully demonstrated the variations in citizens' perspectives on the state in each country during the critical crisis of COVID-19, which will undoubtedly stimulate future research in this area.

Acknowledgment

The research in this chapter was supported by the Japan Society for the Promotion of Science (JSPS) Grants-in-Aid for Scientific Research [grant number 20H00061] and Murata Scientific Foundation.

Notes

1 Other leading approaches include private ownership through division of goods and rule formation through consensus in the community. In the case of COVID-19, however, division of goods is impossible. Community self-governance is partially possible within a narrow scope, but it is still difficult to prevent the spread of an epidemic throughout society.
2 There has been some debate over whether authoritarian or democratic regimes are more efficient in preventing the transmission of COVID-19 over these restrictions on freedom (Annaka, 2021; Cassan and Steenvoort, 2021; Sorci et al., 2020). However, this is not the purpose of the current chapter and is therefore omitted.
3 www.worldvaluessurvey.org/WVSContents.jsp, last viewed June 17, 2024.

References

Annaka, Susumu. 2021. Political regime, data transparency, and COVID-19 death cases. *SSM Population Health* 15: 100832.

Baekgaard, Martin, Julian Christensen, Jonas Krogh Madsen, and Kim Sass Mikkelsen. 2020. Rallying around the flag in times of Covid-19: Societal lockdown and trust in democratic institutions. *Journal of Behavioral Public Administration* 3(2): 1–12.

Cassan, Guilhem and Milan Van Steenvoort. 2021. Political regime and COVID-19 death rate: Efficient, biasing or simply different autocracies?An econometric analysis. *SSM Population Health* 16: 100912.

Cato, Susumu, Takashi Iida, Kenji Ishida, Asei Ito, Kenneth Mori McElwin, and Masahiro Shoji. 2020. Social distancing as a public good under the COVID-19 pandemic. *Public Health* 188: 51–53.

Dalton, Russell and Doh Chull Shin (eds.). 2006. *Citizens, Democracy, and Markets around the Pacific Rim: Congruence Theory and Political Culture*. Oxford: Oxford University Press.

Dalton, Russell J., and Nhu-Ngoc T. Ong., 2005. Authority orientations and democratic attitudes: A test of the "Asian Values" hypothesis. *Japanese Journal of Political Science* 6(2): 211–231.

Dominik, Schraff. 2021. Political trust during the Covid-19 pandemic: Rally around the flag or lockdown effects? *European Journal of Political Research* 60: 1007–1017.

Fukuyama, Francis. 1995. Confucianism and democracy. *Journal of Democracy* 6(2): 20–33.

Gollwitzer, Anton, Cameron Martel, William J. Brady, Philip Pärnamets, Isaac G. Freedman, Eric D. Knowles, and Jay J. van Bavel. 2020. Partisan differences in physical distancing are linked to health outcomes during the COVID-19 pandemic. *Nature Human Behaviour* 4: 1186–1197.

Harvey, David. 2005. *A Brief History of Neoliberalism*. Oxford: Oxford University Press.

Hawkins, Kirk A., Madeleine Read, and Teun Pauwels. 2017. Populism and its causes. In Cristóbal Rovira Kaltwasser, Paul Taggart, Paulina Ochoa Espejo, and Pierre Ostiguy (eds.), *The Oxford Handbook of Populism*. Oxford: Oxford University Press, pp. 267–286.

Hegewald, Sven, and Dominik Sharaff, 2024, Who rallies around the flag?: Evidence from panel data during the Covid-19 pandemic. *Journal of Elections, Public Opinion and Parties*, 34(1): 158–179.

Ikeda, Ken'ichi, 2021, Ajian barometa chosa de shiru 21 seiki no nihon to ajia: Tozai no bunki ten toshite no nihon [Understanding 21st-century Japan and Asia Through the Asian barometer survey: Japan as a crossroads between east and west]. In Ken'ichi Ikeda (ed.) *Nihon to Ajia no Minshushugi o Hakaru*: *Asian Barometer Chosa to Nihon no 21 Seiki* [*Measuring Democracy in Japan and Asia*: *The Asian Barometer Survey and Japan in the 21st Century*] Tokyo: Keiso Shobo, 1–37.

Kerr, John, Costas Panagopoulos, and Sander van der Linden. 2021. Political polarization on COVID-19 pandemic response in the United States. *Personality and Individual Differences* 179: 110892.

Kikkawa, Toru, 2014, *Gendai Nihon no "Shakai no Kokoro": Keiryo Shakai Ishikiron* [*Sociological Social Psychology in Contemporary Japan: Literacy, Consummatory and Reflection*]. Tokyo: Yuhikaku.

Kim, So Young, 2010. Do Asian values exist?: Empirical tests of the four dimensions of Asian values. *Journal of East Asian Studies* 10(2): 315–344.

Marti'nez, De´borah, Cristina Parilli, Carlos Scartascini, and Alberto Simpser. 2021. Let's (not) get together! The role of social norms on social distancing during COVID-19. *PLoS ONE* 16(3): e0247454. https://doi.org/10.1371/journal.pone.0247454.

Matsutani, Mitsuru. 2014. Doshite "shakai wa kaerarenai" noka? [Why "society cannnot be changed?"]. In Naoki Sudo (ed.), *Shakai Ishiki kara Mita Nihon* [*Japan from the Viewpoint of Social Consciousness*]. Tokyo: Yuhikaku, pp. 144–166.

Mudde, Cas and Cristóbal Rovira Kaltwasser. 2017. *Populism*: *A Very Short Introduction*. Oxford: Oxford University Press.

Neville, Fergus G., Anne Templeton, Joanne R. Smith, and Winnifred R. Louis. 2021. Social norms, social identities and the COVID-19 pandemic: Theory and recommendations. *Social and Personality Psychology Compass* 15(5): Article e12596.

Park, Chong Min and Doh Chull Shin. 2006. Do Asian values deter popular support for democracy in South Korea? *Asian Survey* 46(3): 341–361.

Schuman, Howard, Lawrence Bobo, and Maria Krysan. 1992. Authoritarianism in the general population: The education interaction hypothesis. *Social Psychology Quarterly* 55(4): 379–387.

Sorci, Gabriele, Bruno Faivre, and Serge Morand. 2020. Why does COVID-19 case fatality rate vary among countries? https://ssrn.com/abstract=3576892.

Steger, Manfred B. and Ravi K. Roy. 2010. *Neoliberalism: A Very Short Introduction*, Oxford: Oxford University Press.

Stubager, Rune. 2008. Education effects on authoritarian–libertarian values: A question of socialization. *The British Journal of Sociology* 59(2): 327–350.

Zakaria, Fareed and Lee Kuan Yew. 1994. Culture is destiny: A conversation with Lee Kuan Yew. *Foreign Affairs*, 73(2): 109–126.

Zhai, Yida. 2016. Do Confucian values deter Chinese citizens' support for democracy? *Politics and Religion* 10: 261–285.

6 Do Values Prioritizing the Group over the Individual Influence East Asian People's Thought about the Role of the State during the Pandemic?

Taisuke Fujita

Introduction

Any policy decision includes a trade-off between the prioritization of individuals or society. The COVID-19 pandemic forced governments across the world to face this type of trade-off. COVID-19 measures such as movement restrictions, the obligation to wear masks, and vaccination recommendations are typical examples. These measures prioritize the goal of society to prevent the increase in COVID-19 infections and deaths over individual liberties. In fact, those measures have caused protests, especially in Western democracies. However, such protests have been fewer in East Asian countries. As long as COVID-19 measures prioritizing society over individuals are (considered) effective, countries that can take such measures are expected to succeed in reducing infections and deaths.

It has been argued, indeed, that East Asian countries have succeeded in preventing infections and deaths from COVID-19 because of cultural values that prioritize the group or nation over the individual (i.e., collectivism). This chapter contributes to this argument in three respects. First, the present chapter examines whether the above causation holds at the individual level in East Asian countries. If this mechanism is confirmed at the individual level in East Asia, we could be more confident in the above argument. Second, the focus of this chapter is the impact of values on popular attitudes toward the state's economic relief payments for individuals during the pandemic. Existing studies have examined the influence of the values on people's attitudes toward restriction measures such as wearing masks, as explained below. However, COVID-19 measures to restrict mobility and slow the spread of COVID-19 have caused severe recessions (Coibion et al., 2020). Thus, state-provided economic relief could be a prerequisite for introducing such mitigating measures. Both behavioral restrictions (such as wearing masks) and economic relief are indispensable for governments' countermeasures against the pandemic. Accordingly, we expect that social values also influence support for economic relief. If these values are also shown to have an impact on economic support during the pandemic, we would have a deeper understanding of the relationship

DOI: 10.4324/9781003495239-8

between social values and mitigation measures to slow the pandemic. Third, in measuring values prioritizing groups over individuals, we employ a question item with the concrete context of the pandemic, in contrast to existing studies that have utilized abstract question items. People would find it easier to understand and answer a question with a concrete context than an abstract one without context. Moreover, we would like to know what people consider under the very situation of the pandemic. Hence, the question item, including the pandemic context, enables us to identify people's opinions more adequately.

The results of this chapter's analyses show that people who hold values prioritizing society or a group are more likely to support economic relief across the three East Asian countries irrespective of the difference in the political regime and the content of the economic relief between the countries. This finding provides an explanation for the success of East Asian countries in mitigating COVID-19 damage as of 2022.

In the next section, after explaining the concepts related to values prioritizing the group over individual liberties, we propose our hypothesis that the values lead to one's support for economic relief during the pandemic and describe the significance of examining the hypothesis. The second section explains the research design of this chapter, and the third section describes the results of the analyses. A discussion of the analyses and the conclusions of this chapter follow in the last section.

Values Prioritizing the Group over the Individual

Existing studies have shown that values related to the trade-off between the rights of individuals and the benefits to society (or groups) influence people's attitudes toward COVID-19 prevention behaviors. Three types of values are related to this trade-off.

The first is collectivism. Collectivism, as a factor at both the group and individual levels, is characterized by prioritizing a group's goals over individual ones. The concept of collectivism emphasizes the interdependence between the self and one's group or community. Those who hold collectivist values place more value on collective goals and are guided more by group norms and traditional authority figures. To reduce the damage caused by COVID-19, government-initiated nonpharmaceutical interventions are critical. The success of interventions depends on citizen's compliance with restrictive policies. As Conway et al. (2006) claim, the social value orientation of individualism/collectivism can greatly impact how a state addresses the inherent tension between collective/public welfare and individual freedom. Indeed, many existing studies in various fields, such as sociology, social and cultural psychology, and public health, have shown that countries, where collectivism is salient, tend to have fewer deaths during the pandemic, and people in those countries are more compliant with prevention measures, such as wearing masks (Cao et al., 2020; Cho et al., 2022; Huang et al., 2022; Leong et al., 2022; Lu et al., 2021; Maaravi et al., 2021; Rajkumar, 2021; Travaglino and Moon, 2021; Webster et al., 2021).

The second value is authoritarianism. Altemeyer (1988) defines authoritarianism as a value consisting of three elements. First, authoritarians adhere to conventional morality and value compliance with social norms. Second, they emphasize deference to authority figures. Third, they legitimize aggression against those who deviate from social norms.[1] Authoritarianism can be considered similar to collectivism. For example, Kemmelmeier et al. (2003: 307) argue that "the authoritarian emphasis on compliance with social norms and deference to in-group authority has its parallel in the collectivist attention to in-group expectations and respect for status and tradition."

The third value is cultural tightness. Cultural tightness refers to strong norms and a low tolerance of deviant behavior, whereas cultural looseness refers to weak norms and a high tolerance of deviant behavior. Gelfand et al. (2011) measured tightness-looseness (the overall strength of social norms and tolerance of deviance) on a 6-item Likert scale that assessed the degree to which social norms are pervasive, clearly defined, and reliably imposed within nations.[2] Tight cultures have fewer cases and deaths than loose cultures do (Gelfand et al., 2021).

The above three values are, thus, similar in that they prioritize the norms and goals of the group over those of individuals. The values (i.e., collectivism, authoritarianism, and cultural tightness) similarly emphasize the prioritization of a group's goals over individual goals, compliance with social norms, and thus intolerance of deviant behavior from social norms. Because COVID-19 measures involve decisions regarding trade-offs between the prioritization of individuals or society, examining the influence of the values is critical.

East Asians have been argued to hold such values. Studies have shown that East Asian cultures emphasize sacrificing self-interests for the benefit of the group and maintaining harmony within the group (Singelis, 1994; Triandis et al., 1988; Triandis and Gelfand, 1998). To take an example in the context of the pandemic, the restrictions imposed by the Japanese government were limited to requests (rather than enforcement with punishment). The government did not adopt blockade measures, such as lockdowns. However, as Mizuno et al. (2020) argue, the Japanese term typically translated as "request" is understood to be taken as a "demand" by Japanese, implying the strong expectation that those asked will obey the directives, although no legal penalties apply, even if the requests are not followed. The distinctiveness of East Asian cultures appears in whether they quit wearing masks, for example. Whereas many in Western countries quit wearing masks as soon as the obligation was lifted; many Chinese and Koran people are reported to continue wearing masks even after their governments lifted the obligations.[3] Additionally, it is well known that the governments of Singapore and China once emphasized "Asian Values," where the rights of the group are prioritized over those of individuals. In addition, East Asian countries (including China, South Korea, and Japan) are reported to have tighter cultures (Gelfand et al., 2011). Moreover, some studies analyzing Asian countries during the pandemic suggest that collectivism may have increased in these countries (Han et al., 2021; Na et al., 2021).

Accordingly, because East Asian people are more likely (than Western people) to hold values emphasizing the norms and goals of the group, they are expected to be more likely to support the government's COVID-19 measures. The present chapter aims to expand the understanding of the relationship between values and people's attitudes toward COVID-19 measures in three respects.

First, the present chapter focuses on the effect of the values on economic relief payments for individuals during the pandemic, whereas existing studies have examined the effect of the values on behavioral restrictions such as mask-wearing. This chapter proposes that values emphasizing the norms and goals of the group could also influence people's approval of economic relief during the pandemic as well as compliance with prevention measures. This is because economic relief is necessary to introduce prevention measures that restrict economic activities. Those who hold values prioritizing the group are expected to approve of economic support in return for people's compliance with the group's norms, such as wearing masks.

Some might counterargue that those who prioritize individual liberty should be more likely to show positive attitudes toward economic support than those who prioritize the group. Whereas the former reluctantly follow prevention measures such as wearing masks, the latter willingly comply with these measures. Thus, those who prioritize individual liberty should believe that economic support should be provided in return for deference to control measures. In contrast, those who prioritize the group do not think that economic support is necessary to compensate for people's compliance. However, providing economic relief to those who prioritize individual liberty indicates that money will be given to those who might not comply with prevention measures. In contrast, economic support for those who prioritize the group leads to payments to those who would comply with prevention measures. Thus, the latter is more effective and can be justified more easily. Accordingly, we expect those who prioritize the group over individual liberties to be more likely to show positive attitudes toward the state's economic support during the pandemic.

Second, this chapter examines whether the values work at the individual level in the three East Asian countries. If we could confirm that cultural values work at the individual level (in addition to the aggregate national level), we could be more confident that East Asian countries succeeded in preventing COVID-19 infections and deaths due to these values.

Third, while many existing studies have focused on the variation between Asia and other regions, this chapter focuses on the variation within East Asian countries. However, as explained in Chapter 1, whereas the East Asian countries seem to be culturally similar, they vary in terms of their political regimes. The three countries are considered to share a Confucian cultural tradition that emphasizes respect for authority and order. On the other hand, while Japan and South Korea are liberal democracies, China holds an authoritarian political regime. Thus, it is worth examining whether diversity exists in the causation of social values within East Asia.

Thus, the chapter proposes the following hypothesis: people in East Asian countries who hold values prioritizing the norms and goals of the group over those of individuals are more likely to approve of COVID-19 economic relief payments for individuals.

Research Design

In this section, we conduct multiple regression analyses to analyze the impact of the values prioritizing the group on popular support for economic relief payments. Through country-by-country statistical analyses, this chapter aims to examine whether people in East Asian countries differ in terms of the relationship between values and support for economic relief.

The dependent variable of this chapter is the support of respondents for economic relief payments to individuals during the pandemic. For the dependent variable, this chapter uses the following item: "How do you rate the following COVID-19 measures by the government?—Government's economic support for individuals and households." The responses are selected from a 5-point scale, from "5 high" to "1 low." Notably, the characteristics of the government's economic support for individuals differ across East Asian countries. On the one hand, in Japan and South Korea, the government gave all citizens the same amount of money for COVID-19 economic relief.[4] On the other hand, in China, the target of the government's economic support (cash stipends) for individuals has not been for all citizens but has been limited to people with low incomes.

With respect to independent variables, as explained above, the values this chapter focuses on (i.e., collectivism, authoritarianism, and cultural tightness) similarly emphasize the prioritization of a group's goals over individual goals, compliance with social norms, and thus intolerance of deviant behavior from social norms. These factors are considered in deciding the question items to measure the values for our independent variables. In addition, the item measuring the values prioritizing the group should focus on the context of the pandemic. Emphasizing the context in the question item has two merits. First, we would like to know people's thoughts in the context of the pandemic. Second, by introducing the concrete context, a respondent would find it easy to choose a response that is the closest to one's actual thought. This merit enables us to grasp a respondent's real thoughts. Therefore, it is better to make a respondent think with the context in mind.

Accordingly, this chapter employs the following two question items for independent variables that measure whether respondents' values prioritize the group. One is "What do you think about the following statements?—We should fully comply with government's anti-pandemic policies, no matter how inconvenient these policies are." Responses are on a 5-point scale. The respondents chose from "5 strongly agree" to "1 strongly disagree." This item aims to grasp whether a respondent prioritizes a group's goals over individual goals and to comply with social norms in the context of the COVID-19 pandemic.

The results of the three East Asian countries are compared in terms of the extent to which people hold values prioritizing the group over individuals at the national level.

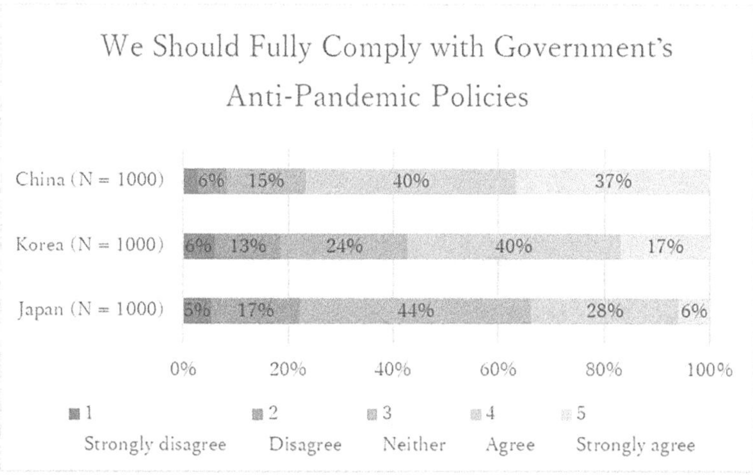

Figure 6.1 Ratios of respondents who approve of values prioritizing the group (compliance).

As Figure 6.1 shows, in the order of China, South Korea, and Japan, people are more likely to agree that "We should fully comply with government anti-pandemic policies." This implies that, in the order of China, South Korea, and Japan, people are more likely to hold the values prioritizing the group over individual liberties.

The other item interrogating an independent variable is "What do you think about following statements on the attitude toward government policies?—In emergencies, every citizen should watch over [their neighbors] to ensure that government policies are respected."[5] Respondents chose from a 5-point scale: "5 strongly agree" to "1 strongly disagree." This item aims to measure the extent to which a respondent prioritizes a group's goals and is intolerant of deviant behaviors.

Figure 6.2 shows a similar pattern to Figure 6.1 in that in the order of China, South Korea, and Japan, people are more likely to agree that "In emergencies, every citizen should watch over [their neighbors] to ensure that government policies are respected."

Irrespective of the indices measuring the values prioritizing the group, the pattern between the countries is similar. While East Asian people are frequently considered to value collectivism, authoritarianism, and cultural tightness, there is a difference in the extent to which people hold such values between the East Asian countries at the national level. Through the following analyses, we examined whether the difference in the values at the national level could also be observed in terms of individual causation.

We included several control variables in the analysis. First, existing studies have shown that concern about COVID-19 affects people's attitudes toward government COVID-19 policies (Jørgensen et al., 2021; Rees-Jones et al., 2022). One would need money when infected with COVID-19, which might require payment for

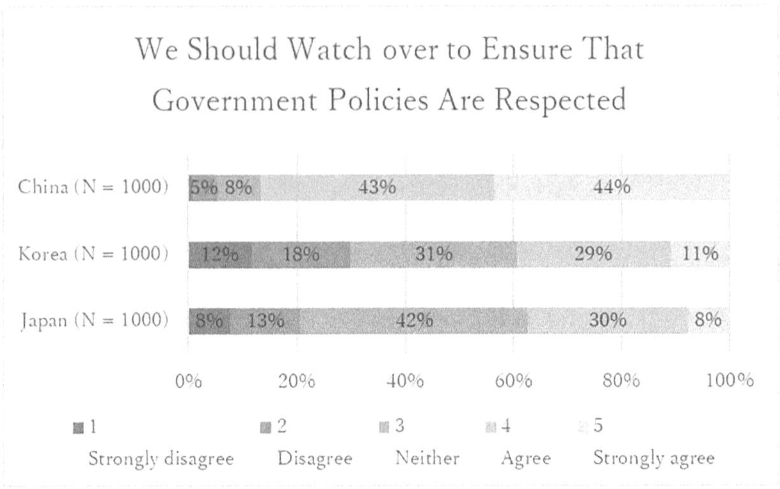

Figure 6.2 Ratios of respondents who approve of values prioritizing the group (tolerance).

treatment and a decrease in one's income. Thus, it is naturally expected that people worried about COVID-19 tend to support the government's policies of economic support.[6]

Second, if one experienced a decrease in income after the pandemic began, he or she is apt to seek government economic support. Accordingly, respondents who faced an income decrease after the pandemic began are more likely to show a positive attitude toward economic support than those who did not.[7]

In addition, we include social demographic variables. The older one is, the more likely one is to approve of economic support. This is because elderly people are more vulnerable to the pandemic in terms of health conditions. Thus, the variable of age is included. The variable of gender is also included, as women are expected to show a positive attitude due to their relatively low income compared with men. Educational background could influence attitudes toward economic support because the policy includes a distributional function even if the amount to be paid is the same for every citizen. Similarly, one's subjective social class could determine one's posture toward the policy. Thus, the greater the educational background and the higher the subjective social class is, the more likely one is to hold a negative attitude toward economic relief. Additionally, the ideological position held by a respondent might be a determinant of one's attitude toward the policy. The more liberal an ideology one holds, the more one supports economic relief. Therefore, the variables of educational background, subjective social class, and ideology are also included in the analysis.

Finally, existing studies have argued that people who support the current ruling party are more likely (than those who do not) to support the government's COVID-19 policy (Altiparmakis et al., 2021; Jørgensen et al., 2021; Yamamoto and Fujita,

2023). This indicates that people approve of economic support during the pandemic not because they have an opinion on the content of the policy but because the policy was decided by a political party that they support. This variable is included in the following analyses of the data for Japan and South Korea, which are democracies.

Results

We run ordinal logistic regression analyses country by country, as the dependent variable is a 5-point scale. Table 6.1 shows the results. The upper number of each cell indicates an odds ratio. The odds ratio is a measure of the association between a cause and an outcome. It represents the odds that the level of an outcome will rise given a particular cause compared with the odds of the outcome occurring given a lower level of the cause. If the odds ratio of a cause is greater than 1.0, the cause has a positive influence on the level of the outcome. In contrast, if the odds ratio of a cause is lower than 1.0, the cause has a negative influence on the level of the outcome.

The left column shows the analysis results for Japanese respondents. Both indices for the values prioritizing the group over individual liberties have a positive effect on support for economic relief payments. People who believe that one should fully comply with government anti-pandemic policies and those who think that every citizen should watch over their neighbors to ensure that government policies are respected are more likely to support economic relief payments during the pandemic. Irrespective of whether the value is measured with a focus on the factor of compliance with authority or a focus on intolerance of deviant behaviors, the values prioritizing the group over individual liberties lead respondents to hold positive postures toward economic relief. In contrast, surprisingly, those suffering income decreases during the pandemic are less likely to show positive attitudes. With the above results considered together, Japanese respondents seem to consider whether they support economic relief from the viewpoint of society or the group rather than that of their own individual condition.

No social demographic variable has a statistically significant effect. Although the variables were expected to have an impact according to existing studies and conventional understanding, that is not the case. This indicates the importance of the values prioritizing the group for Japanese respondents as determinants of people's preference for economic relief during the pandemic.[8]

The middle column of Table 6.1 shows the results of the analysis of survey data in South Korea. Both indices of the values prioritizing the group over individual liberties have a positive effect on support for economic relief payments, as they do in Japan. South Korean respondents are also similar to Japanese respondents in that the experience of a decrease in income leads to a negative attitude toward economic relief.

In contrast to Japanese respondents, some sociodemographic variables have a statistically significant influence on South Korean respondents. Conservative ideology, high educational background, and high subjective social class lead to a negative attitude toward economic relief, in line with our expectations. Variables

Table 6.1 Ordinal logistic analysis of people's support for economic relief payments during the pandemic in East Asian countries

	Japan	*South Korea*	*China*
Age	1.00	1.01	1.00
	(0.99–1.00)	(1.00–1.01)	(0.99–1.01)
Female	1.04	0.87	1.48***
	(0.80–1.34)	(0.69–1.09)	(1.15–1.91)
Class	0.89	0.80***	0.82***
	(0.77–1.04)	(0.70–0.92)	(0.71–0.95)
Infection	1.00	1.00	0.99
	(0.99–1.00)	(1.00–1.00)	(0.94–1.04)
Conservative	1.05	0.86***	0.93**
	(0.95–1.16)	(0.78–0.94)	(0.88–1.00)
Education	1.02	0.80*	0.74**
	(0.77–1.34)	(0.63–1.01)	(0.55–1.00)
COVID_econhard	0.65***	0.87**	0.82***
	(0.54–0.77)	(0.76–0.98)	(0.73–0.92)
VALUE_comply	1.73***	1.49***	1.77***
	(1.49–2.01)	(1.32–1.69)	(1.55–2.02)
VALUE_watchover	1.40***	1.24***	1.56***
	(1.22–1.61)	(1.11–1.38)	(1.34–1.82)
Observations	813	958	1000

Note: The table presents the odds ratios and lower and upper confidence limit (in parentheses) from the ordinal logistic regression.
* $p < .10$, ** $p < .05$, *** $p < .01$.

such as age, gender, and concern about COVID-19 infection are not determinants of people's preference for economic support, even in South Korea.[9]

The right column of Table 6.1 shows the analysis results for the Chinese respondents. As in both Japanese and Korean respondents, while the indices of the values prioritizing the group over individual liberties have a positive effect on support for economic relief payments, the decrease in income during the pandemic has a negative effect on attitudes toward economic relief.

Social demographic variables, such as conservative ideology, high educational background, and high subjective social class, lead Chinese respondents to show a negative attitude toward economic support, as we observed in the analysis of South Korean data. In contrast to the gender variable in South Korea, gender has a statistically significant effect in China. Women are more likely to have a positive attitude toward economic relief payments.

By comparing the results of the above analyses, we can identify both common and differing features between the East Asian countries. On the one hand, there is a difference in the ratio of those who hold values prioritizing the group over individual liberties at the national level (Figures 6.1 and 6.2). In the order of China, South Korea, and Japan, people are more likely to prioritize the group. On the other hand, it is common at the individual level among the three countries that the values prioritizing the group over individual liberties caused a positive posture toward economic relief during the pandemic (Table 6.1). We observe these relationships irrespective of the indices measuring values for group priority over individual liberties.

Discussion and Conclusion

Do the values prioritizing the group over individual liberties determine people's attitudes toward economic relief payments during the pandemic? At the national level, the three countries differ in the extent to which people hold values prioritizing the group. In the order of China, South Korea, and Japan, people are more likely to prioritize the group first. At the individual level, our hypothesis that collectivist values lead to support for economic relief is supported similarly in all three countries. Those who approve of values emphasizing norm compliance and group goals are more likely to show positive attitudes toward economic relief payments (than those who do not approve of the values).

In interpreting the results, we should note that the East Asian countries vary in important respects. While Japan and South Korea are democracies, China is not. Whereas Japan and South Korea have provided economic relief payments to all citizens with the same amount of money irrespective of economic conditions such as income, China has limited the target of payments according to the recipients' economic conditions. Nevertheless, these collectivist values have a similar positive effect on support for economic relief across all East Asian countries. Furthermore, in the analysis of Japanese data, no variables other than collectivist values have a statistically significant effect on support for economic relief. Therefore, we can conclude that the values prioritizing the group are critical determinants of support for the state's economic role.

Studies have shown that people in East Asian countries are more likely to hold values prioritizing the group over individual liberties than are those in Western countries at the national level. In addition, studies have demonstrated that values such as collectivism and cultural tightness positively influence people's compliance with mitigation measures such as wearing masks, which has successfully reduced COVID-19 damage.

This chapter contributes to the understanding of East Asian countries' success in mitigating COVID-19 damage as of 2022 by adding new findings about the influence of collectivist values on COVID-19 measures. We have shown at the individual level that people in East Asian countries who approve of values prioritizing the group are more likely (than those who do not approve) to approve of economic relief, which is a prerequisite for introducing mitigating measures that restrict individual liberty, such as restricting mobility and wearing masks. Accordingly, the values prioritizing groups have an impact on the reduction in infections and deaths caused by COVID-19 not only through high compliance with behavioral restrictions, which has been the focus of existing studies. The values might have contributed to the reduction through the approval of economic relief, which is the prerequisite of behavioral restrictions. Hence, on the basis of the individual-level analysis, East Asian success with COVID-19 measures is partly due to the number of people who approve of COVID-19 mitigation measures due to values that prioritize the group. Therefore, East Asian countries naturally succeeded in implementing COVID-19 countermeasures because of their citizens' values.

We admit that the findings of this chapter have external validity problems in terms of time. The COVID-19 conditions in East Asian countries have come closer to those in Western countries since the survey was conducted at the beginning of 2022 for this book's project. In East Asian countries, COVID-19-related damage, such as the number of infections and deaths, has increased. China terminated its "zero-COVID" policy in January 2023. This change in COVID-19 conditions in East Asian countries might influence people's preference for COVID-19 measures. People might have responded differently if the survey was conducted in 2023. We need to conduct additional surveys to determine whether the findings of this chapter (the effects of the values prioritizing group) are robust.

Acknowledgment

This research was supported by the Japan Society for the Promotion of Science (JSPS) Grants-in-Aid for Scientific Research [grant number 20H00061], Murata Scientific Foundation, and the Nagasaki University State of the Art Research program.

Notes

1 Some studies argue that authoritarian states have succeeded in preventing COVID-19 (Sorci et al., 2020; Cassan and Steenvoort, 2021; Narita and Sudo, 2021). However, some studies call for attention to the fact that public data in authoritarian states lack transparency (Cassan and Steenvoort, 2021; Annaka, 2021).

2 The six scale items are as follows. (1) There are many social norms that people are supposed to abide by in this country. (2) In this country, there are very clear expectations for how people should act in most situations. (3) People in this country agree on what behaviors are appropriate versus inappropriate in most situations. (4) People in this country have a great deal of freedom in deciding how they want to behave in most situations. (5) In this country, if someone acts in an inappropriate way, others will strongly disapprove. (6) People in this country almost always comply with social norms.

3 "National characteristics appear whether people quit wearing masks," *Nihon Keizai Shimbun*, February 4, 2023.

4 In Japan, the government provided all citizens with 100,000 yen (approximately 1000 $USD at the exchange rate in 2020). In South Korea, the government gave all citizens 250,000 won (230 $USD at the exchange rate in 2020) twice in 2020 and 2021.

5 This question item is employed by Miura et al. (2020), which aims to measure the obedience to social norms.

6 The wording of the question item for this variable is as follows. "How likely do you think the following situation is to happen? In a year's time, you will get infected by the Coronavirus (COVID-19) and be hospitalized. Please answer an approximate number."

7 The wording of the question item for this variable is "What do you think about the situation around you after the coronavirus pandemic began?" The response choices are a

little different between the countries. In China, after reading "I and/or any of my family experienced a decrease in income due to the Coronavirus (COVID-19) pandemic," respondents chose from "1 not at all" to "5 very much." In Japan and Korea, respondents read "After the pandemic began, your income and your household's income ..." and chose from "1 A increased," "2 close to A," "3 Neither A nor B," "4 close to B," "5 B decreased."

8 If we included the variable of government political party support in the analyses, the variable has a statistically significant effect as existing studies have shown. Those who support the ruling government party are more likely to support economic relief. However, the inclusion of the variable does not change the results of which variables have statistically significant influence in which direction.

9 If we included the variable of government political party support in the analyses, the variable has statistically significant effect as it does in the analysis of Japanese respondents. Including the variable does not change the above results.

References

Altemeyer, Bob. 1988. *Enemies of Freedom: Understanding Right-Wing Authoritarianism.* San Francisco: Jossey-Bass.

Altiparmakis, Argyrios, Abel Bojar, Sylvain Brouard, Martial Foucault, Hanspeter Kriesi, and Richard Nadeau. 2021. Pandemic politics: Policy evaluations of government responses to Covid-19. *West European Politics* 44(5–6): 1159–1179.

Annaka, Susumu. 2021. Political regime, data transparency, and COVID-19 deaths cases. *SSM-Population Health* 15: 100832.

Cao, Cong, Ning Li, and Li Liu. 2020. Do national cultures matter in the containment of COVID-19? *International Journal of Sociology and Social Policy* 40(9/10): 939–961.

Cassan, Guilhem, and Milan Van Steenvoort. 2021. Political regime and COVID 19 death rate: Efficient, biasing or simply different? Autocracies? An econometric analysis. *SSM-Population Health* 16: 100912.

Cho, Hyewon, Yafei Guo, and Carlos Torelli. 2022. Collectivism fosters preventive behaviors to contain the spread of COVID-19: Implications for social marketing in public health. *Psychology & Marketing* 39(4): 694–700.

Coibion, Olivier, Yuriy Gorodnichenko, and Michael Weber. 2020. The cost of the COVID-19 crisis: Lockdowns, macroeconomic expectations, and consumer spending. National Bureau of Economic Research, working paper 27141. DOI: 10.3386/w27141.

Conway III, Lucian Gideon, Shannon M Sexton, and Roger G Tweed. 2006. Collectivism and governmentally initiated restrictions: A cross-sectional and longitudinal analysis across nations and within a nation. *Journal of Cross-Cultural Psychology* 37(1): 20–41.

Gelfand, Michele J, Jana L Raver, Lisa Nishii, Lisa M Leslie, Janetta Lun, Beng Chong Lim, Lili Duan, *et al.* 2011. Differences between tight and loose cultures: A 33-nation study. *Science* 332(6033): 1100–1104.

Gelfand, Michele J, Joshua Conrad Jackson, Xinyue Pan, Dana Nau, Dylan Pieper, Emmy Denison, Munqith Dagher, *et al.* 2021. The relationship between cultural tightness–looseness and Covid-19 cases and deaths: A global analysis. *The Lancet Planetary Health* 5(3): e135–e44.

Han, Nuo, Xiaopeng Ren, Peijing Wu, Xiaoqian Liu, and Tingshao Zhu. 2021. Increase of collectivistic expression in China during the Covid-19 outbreak: An empirical study on online social networks. *Frontiers in Psychology* 12: 632204.

Huang, Li, Oliver Zhen Li, Baiqiang Wang, and Zilong Zhang. 2022. Individualism and the fight against Covid-19. *Humanities and Social Sciences Communications* 9: 120.

Jørgensen, Frederik, Alexander Bor, Marie Fly Lindholt, and Michael Bang Petersen. 2021. Public support for government responses against Covid-19: Assessing levels and predictors in eight Western democracies during 2020. *West European Politics* 44(5–6): 1129–1158.

Kemmelmeier, Markus, Eugene Burnstein, Krum Krumov, Petia Genkova, Chie Kanagawa, Matthew S Hirshberg, Hans-Peter Erb, Grazyna Wieczorkowska, and Kimberly A Noels. 2003. Individualism, collectivism, and authoritarianism in seven societies. *Journal of Cross-Cultural Psychology* 34(3): 304–322.

Leong, Suyi, Kimin Eom, Keiko Ishii, Marion C. Aichberger, Karolina Fetz, Tim S. Müller, Heejung S. Kim, and David K. Sherman. 2022. Individual costs and community benefits: Collectivism and individuals' compliance with public health interventions. *PLoS One* 17(11): e0275388.

Lu, Jackson G., Peter Jin, and Alexander S. English. 2021. Collectivism predicts mask use during Covid-19. *Proceedings of the National Academy of the Sciences* 118(23): e2021793118.

Maaravi, Yossi, Aharon Levy, Tamar Gur, Dan Confino, and Sandra Segal. 2021. "The tragedy of the commons": How individualism and collectivism affected the spread of the Covid-19 pandemic. *Frontiers in Public Health* 9: 627559.

Miura, Asako, Kai Hiraishi, Daisuke Nakanishi, and Andrea Ortolani. 2020. International Comparative Analysis of Attitudes toward COVID-19 Infection Disaster: Are "Getting One's Just Deserts" and "Coronavirus Vigilantes" Unique to Japan? [Shingata Korona-Uirusu Kansenka Ni Taisuru Taido no Kokusai Hikaku: "Jigou-jitoku" "Jishuku-keisatsu" Ha Nihon Ni Yuniiku Nanoka]. *Proceedings of the 61st conference of the Japanese Society of Social Psychology*, November 7–8, 2020.

Mizuno, Masafumi, Chiyo Fujii, and Tsutomu Sakuta. 2020. The Covid-19 pandemic and social psychiatry: Lessons shared, lessons learned—a Japanese perspective. *World Social Psychiatry* 2(2): 134.

Na, Jinkyung, Namhee Kim, Hye Won Suk, Eunsoo Choi, Jong An Choi, Joo Hyun Kim, Soolim Kim, and Incheol Choi. 2021. Individualism-collectivism during the Covid-19 pandemic: A field study testing the pathogen stress hypothesis of individualism-collectivism in Korea. *Personality and Individual Differences* 183: 111127.

Narita, Yusuke, and Ayumi Sudo. 2021. Curse of democracy: Evidence from 2020. Available at SSRN 3827327.

Oyserman, Daphna, Heather M Coon, and Markus Kemmelmeier. 2002. Rethinking individualism and collectivism: Evaluation of theoretical assumptions and meta-analyses. *Psychological Bulletin* 128(1): 3–72.

Rajkumar, Ravi Philip. 2021. The relationship between measures of individualism and collectivism and the impact of Covid-19 across nations. *Public Health in Practice* 2: 100143.

Rees-Jones, Alex, John D'Attoma, Amedeo Piolatto, and Luca Salvadori. 2022. Experience of the Covid-19 pandemic and support for safety-net expansion. *Journal of Economic Behavior & Organization* 200: 1090–1104.

Singelis, Theodore M. 1994. The measurement of independent and interdependent self-construals. *Personality and Social Psychology Bulletin* 20(5): 580–591.

Sorci, Gabriele, Bruno Faivre, and Serge Morand. 2020. Why does COVID-19 case fatality rate vary among countries? *Scientific Reports* 10: 18909.

Travaglino, Giovanni A, and Chanki Moon. 2021. Compliance and self-reporting during the Covid-19 pandemic: A cross-cultural study of trust and self-conscious emotions in the United States, Italy, and South Korea. *Frontiers in Psychology* 12: 565845.

Triandis, Harry C. 1989. The self and social behavior in differing cultural contexts. *Psychological Review* 96(3): 506–520.

Triandis, Harry C, and Michele J Gelfand. 1998. Converging measurement of horizontal and vertical individualism and collectivism. *Journal of Personality and Social Psychology* 74(1): 118–128.

Triandis, Harry C, Robert Bontempo, Marcelo J Villareal, Masaaki Asai, and Nydia Lucca. 1988. Individualism and collectivism: Cross-cultural perspectives on self-ingroup relationships. *Journal of Personality and Social Psychology* 54(2): 323–338.

Webster, Gregory D, Jennifer L Howell, Joy E Losee, Elizabeth A Mahar, and Val Wongsomboon. 2021. Culture, Covid-19, and collectivism: A paradox of American exceptionalism? *Personality and Individual Differences* 178: 110853.

Yamamoto, Hidehiro and Taisuke Fujita. 2023. State-society relations under the COVID disaster in Japan. In Jozef Oleński, Jeffrey Sachs, Masayuki Susai, Yannis Tsekouras, and Arjan Gjonça (eds.), *Handbook of Research on Socio-Economic Sustainability in the Post-Pandemic Era*. Hershey: IGI Global, pp.139–157.

7 Does Rawls' Perspective Influence East Asian People's Thinking about the Role of the State during the Pandemic?

Taisuke Fujita

Introduction

COVID-19 has expanded the role of states across the world. Governments have restricted individuals' liberty by restricting their movement, demanding that people wear masks, and requesting that people be vaccinated. Moreover, governments have increased their expenditures by providing economic support for households and businesses. The state's role has been inevitable in attempts to decrease infections and deaths caused by COVID-19 and to alleviate the economic damage to individuals caused by COVID-19, at least to some extent. Thus, have people's expectations of the state's role changed throughout the pandemic? The present chapter focuses on economic relief payments for individuals and households during the pandemic. This research question is essential in considering the state's role after the pandemic. Furthermore, focusing on this policy is fruitful because it resembles universal basic income (UBI) in Japan and Korea, as benefits of the same amount were paid to all the people/households in the countries irrespective of the recipients' economic conditions. Thus, the analyses will also enable us to infer people's preferences for UBI after the pandemic.

This chapter explores the above research question from Rawls's perspective, which emphasizes the role of luck in one's achievements, such as income. As explained below, existing studies have shown that one's perception of the extent to which people control their own fate is a critical determinant of attitudes toward redistribution policies, for example. Accordingly, investigating whether the perception of the role of luck influences people's support for the policy of economic support during the pandemic is fruitful. Given that people's perceptions of the impact of luck determine their support for redistribution, analyzing the relationship between people's perceptions of luck and people's attitudes toward economic relief payments during the pandemic hints at whether people are likely to accept the expansion of the government's economic role after the pandemic.

The results of our analyses indicate that Japanese and Koreans who believe that luck affects people's achievement tend to have positive attitudes toward orthodox redistribution, which existing studies have found for Westerners. However, Japanese, Korean, and Chinese people who consider the economic damage caused by the pandemic to be due to bad luck are less likely to have positive attitudes

DOI: 10.4324/9781003495239-9

toward economic support policies during the pandemic. These results imply that the pandemic has not changed people's expectations about the role of the state. That is, the expansion of the state's economic role is unlikely to be realized.

The following section explains why this chapter focuses on the impact of luck on the basis of existing studies and shows the variation in the perception of luck among the three East Asian countries. After the characteristics of economic relief payments during the pandemic are explained in the second section, we introduce the research question of this chapter in the third section and explain the research design in the fourth section. Then, we present the results of our analyses. Finally, in the last section, we present a discussion and conclusion.

Rawls' Perspective and the State's Economic Support during the Pandemic

Who supported the economic relief payments made by the state for individuals during the COVID-19 pandemic? In considering what roles the state should assume, the attitude toward luck is an important determinant. Rawls (1971) argues that the benefit to the least well-off should be maximized according to the "maximin principle"—the decision principle that maximizes the minimum outcome. This argument is based on the thought experiment of the "veil of ignorance." By wearing a veil of ignorance, we cannot know who we are and cannot identify our personal circumstances, such as family background, talent, and others. By being ignorant of our circumstances, we can more objectively consider how societies should operate. Rawls (1971), Sandel (2007, 2020), and others argue that inequality due to family background, talent, or opportunities results from luck.[1] Thus, in a just society, the effect of luck should be minimized.[2] Indeed, existing behavioral studies have included empirical experiments that examine whether the thought experiment proposed by Rawls is valid and demonstrate that such concerns about minimums may operate as a strong psychological anchor in social distributions (Frohlich and Oppenheimer, 1992; Engelmann and Strobel, 2004; Norton and Ariely, 2011). Some have criticized that their empirical experimental results are invalid, as the "veil of ignorance" cannot be realized. However, Kameda et al. (2016) show that social distribution for others is psychologically linked to risky decision-making (such as gambling) for the self. That is, the factor of luck plays a role in people's thinking about social distribution.

Accordingly, if people perceive that luck (which cannot be controlled by one's effort) influences one's situation, such as being rich/poor or successful/a failure, one might consider that the influence of luck should be alleviated by the state's policy. Existing studies indeed have shown that differences in perceptions of luck lead to differences in attitudes toward redistribution policies among people in different countries. For example, Bénabou and Tirole (2016) noted that the World Values Survey shows considerable differences in beliefs about the role of effort versus luck in life. In the United States, approximately 60% of people believe that effort is key, whereas in Western Europe, only 30% do so on average. In addition, these nationally dominant beliefs have little relationship with the facts about social mobility or how much those living in poverty work. Nevertheless, they are strongly correlated with the share of social spending in GDP (Alesina, Glaeser, and Sacerdote, 2001). Even at the individual level, voters' perceptions of the extent to which people control their own fate are critical determinants of attitudes toward inequality and redistribution (Fong, 2001).

Attitudes toward the role of luck may influence what individuals think of the state's measures against the COVID-19 pandemic, as they influence whether people approve of orthodox redistribution policies. As Figure 7.1 shows, in Japan and Korea, approximately half of the respondents agreed that "If the new coronavirus pandemic negatively influenced anyone's employment or income, I think it was due to his or her bad luck." In contrast, only approximately 20% of the Chinese respondents thought that the pandemic's negative impact on one's economic situation was due to bad luck, whereas approximately 40% of the Chinese respondents thought that the impact was due to factors that fell under one's own responsibility. Those in the three countries that consider economic damage during the pandemic to be due to bad luck might support a policy of economic support by the government during the pandemic.

Moreover, there are apparent differences in people's perceptions of luck among East Asian countries, as our analysis shows below. We conducted multiple correspondence analysis to check the variation in attitudes toward luck between the countries. By checking the multiple-dimensional patterns regarding luck, we gained a general understanding of the differences in attitudes toward luck among the countries. In the analysis, we used the responses to the following question items related to attitudes toward luck.

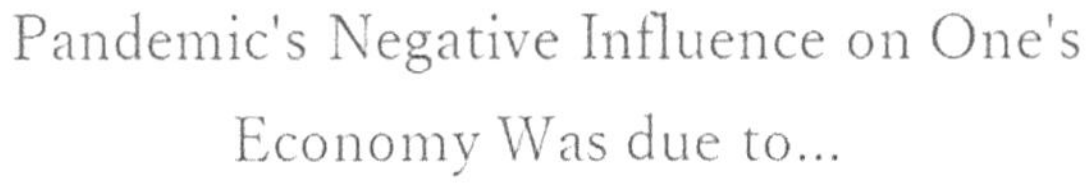

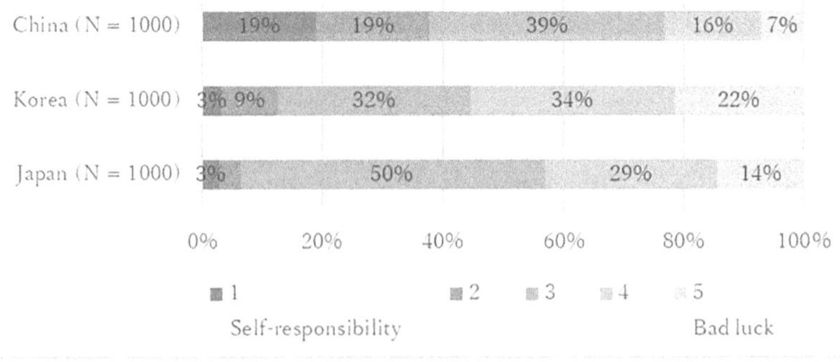

Figure 7.1 Ratios of people's thoughts about the cause of the pandemic's negative influence on individual economic conditions.

[COVID_infection_luck] Respondents read the following prompt: "Regarding the damage caused by COVID-19, there are two contrasting views, A and B. With which of the views do you agree? If anyone was infected with the new coronavirus, I think it was due to ..." Then, they chose from "1 A his or her self-responsibility," "2 close to A," "3 Neither A nor B," "4 close to B," and "5 B his or her bad luck."

[COVID_economy_luck] Respondents read the following prompt: "Regarding the damage caused by COVID-19, there are two contrasting views, A and B. With which of the views do you agree? If anyone's employment or income was negatively impacted by the new coronavirus pandemic, I think it was due to ..." Then, they chose from "1 A his or her self-responsibility," "2 close to A," "3 Neither A nor B," "4 close to B," and "5 B his or her bad luck."

[STATUS_luck] "How much do you agree or disagree with the following statement? One's social status is determined by the wealth of one's family growing up." Respondents chose an answer from a 5-point scale ranging from "5 strongly agree" to "1 strongly disagree."

[POOR_luck] "How much do you agree or disagree with the following statement? If anyone is poor, I think it is due to his or her bad luck." Respondents chose an answer from a 5-point scale ranging from "5 strongly agree" to "1 strongly disagree."

Figure 7.2 shows the results of multiple correspondence analysis. For the analysis, we simplified the 5-point scale to a 3-point scale. We combined the original "1" and "2" ratings into a new "1," kept the original "3" as "2," and merged the original "4" and "5" ratings into a new "3." In Korea, Japan, and China, in that order, people consider luck to determine what one achieves. More specifically, Korean respondents were most likely to choose answer "3" to all the questions, indicating that they consider luck to play a role in one's outcomes, such as one's social status and whether one faces negative economic impacts due to the pandemic. In contrast, Chinese respondents tended to choose "1" consistently, implying that Chinese people do not believe that luck is an important determinant of one's outcomes. Japanese respondents chose "2" most often, indicating that their way of thinking lies somewhere between that of Koreans and Chinese. The above results suggest that the attitude toward luck varies across East Asian countries and that the pattern of the variation is stable across the different question items regarding the role of luck. We analyze whether people's perceptions of the influence of luck on their support for economic relief also differ across countries at the individual level.

Characteristics of Economic Relief Payments during the Pandemic

Have people's thoughts about the state's role changed throughout the pandemic? While numerous studies have examined changes in social policy preferences during the pandemic, their conclusions are mixed. For example, Daniele et al. (2020) reported that respondents to a survey under COVID-19 treatment became less supportive of taxation to pay for welfare policies in Germany, the Netherlands,

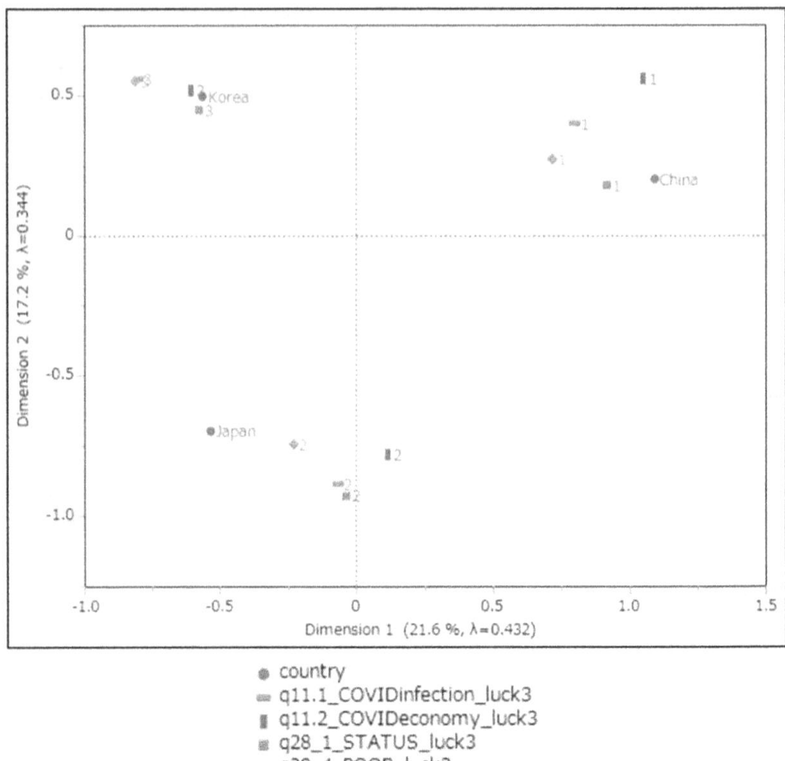

Figure 7.2 Patterns in attitudes toward luck (multiple correspondence analysis).

Italy, and Spain. In contrast, Klemm and Mauro (2022) reported increasing support for progressive taxation in the United States. Analyzing panel data from Germany, Sweden, and Spain, Ares et al. (2021) reported no change in the levels of support for redistribution before and after the pandemic began. In addition, Blumenau et al. (2021), using British panel data, and Reeskens et al. (2021), analyzing Dutch panel data, found no evidence that preferences for redistribution increased from pre-pandemic levels.

The studies above analyzed people's attitudes toward the same policy, the orthodox redistribution policy, before and after the pandemic began to examine whether people's preferences changed throughout the pandemic. In analyzing people's preferences regarding redistribution policies, however, we should bear in mind that the structure of economic relief payments during the pandemic differed from that of orthodox redistribution policies. Most redistribution policies give recipients different amounts of money according to their economic conditions, such as their income. In contrast, the most common financial support policy for individuals during the pandemic in Japan and Korea (but not in China) was that the same amount of money was paid to all the people, irrespective of their income.[3] Hence, economic support during the pandemic in Japan and Korea has resembled UBI, which is a fixed amount paid to all individuals without testing or work requirements (Van Parijs, 2004). Thus, we must consider certain differences when investigating changes in people's preferences.

With respect to people's preference for UBI, Nettle et al. (2021) reported that "people expressed much stronger support for a UBI policy for the times of the pandemic and its aftermath than for normal times." Weisstanner (2022) reported that younger and poorer people are more likely to support UBI. Additionally, while women in general are more likely to oppose UBI, respondents who hold a left-wing ideology are more supportive of UBI. This division regarding attitudes toward UBI has been maintained during the pandemic. To gain a better understanding of whether and why people have begun to support UBI throughout the pandemic, it is reasonable to compare people's preferences for economic relief, which is similar to UBI, and for orthodox redistribution policies.[4] This is what this chapter addresses.

Research Question

Thus, the present chapter investigates the impact of people's attitudes toward luck on their support for economic relief payments provided by the state during the COVID-19 pandemic. As the attitude toward luck determines people's approval of orthodox redistribution policies, the more people consider the achievements of people to be due to luck, the more they might approve of economic support during the pandemic. Is this the case? Alternatively, do people show different attitudes toward orthodox redistribution and economic relief policies during the pandemic?

In addition, there might be differences in attitudes among East Asian countries. For example, Osberg and Smeeding (2006) reported that Americans were less concerned about economic inequality than citizens from other nations were. Do attitudes toward luck influence whether people in East Asia approve of state measures regarding economic relief? This chapter aims to expand our understanding of people's preferences regarding the state's role in that our focus is a comparison among East Asian countries. Many existing studies have focused on Western countries such as the US and EU countries. However, findings in Western countries do not necessarily apply to East Asian countries. Moreover, variations among East Asian countries have rarely been explored.

Research Design

This chapter aims to answer the following two research questions: (1) Do people's beliefs about luck's role determine their support for economic relief payments during the pandemic as well as orthodox redistribution policies? (2) Is there a difference between East Asian countries in the influence of people's thoughts about luck on their support for the state's economic role in such policies? To answer these questions, this chapter includes the following analyses. First, we run multiple regression analyses country by country to check whether people's perceptions of the role of luck impact their preferences regarding the state's economic policies, orthodox redistribution policies, and economic relief payments made during the pandemic. If their perception of luck impacts their beliefs about economic relief in the same way it does their beliefs about orthodox redistribution, this implies that people view COVID-19 economic relief as an extension of orthodox redistribution. Second, we compare the results of the regression analyses among countries. If the results regarding the impact of the perception of luck differ, we can see that the influence of beliefs about the role of luck is not universal. It might be that Rawls's argument is valid only for certain countries.

We now explain the measurement of variables for the following regression analyses. The dependent variables in this chapter are respondents' support for orthodox redistribution policies and economic relief payments for individuals and households during the pandemic. For these variables, we use the following question items.

[Orthodox redistribution policy] What do you think about the following statements about the state's role? "The government has a responsibility to take care of people who can't care for themselves." Respondents responded on a 5-point scale ranging from "5 strongly agree" to "1 strongly disagree."

[Economic relief during the pandemic] "How do you rate the success of the following COVID-19 measures by the government?—Government's economic support for individuals and households." The responses were given on a 5-point scale ranging from "5 high" to "1 low."

The independent variable measures a respondent's perception of the importance of luck as a determinant of achievement, such as one's economic situation (i.e., income). We use two questions for the independent variable. To analyze the determinants of people's support for orthodox redistribution policies, we use the following item: [POOR_luck]. We chose this item for two reasons. First, Rawls emphasized the benefit to the least well-off. Thus, selecting an item focused on those living in poverty should be valid. Second, the question item for the dependent variable concerns economic support for those living in poverty. Therefore, the item best corresponds to the dependent variable.

[POOR_luck] "How much do you agree or disagree with the following statement? If anyone is poor, I think it is due to his or her bad luck." Respondents choose their answer on a 5-point scale ranging from "5 strongly agree" to "1 strongly disagree."

In contrast, when we examine determinants of people's support for economic relief payments during the pandemic, we use the following item: [COVID_economy_luck]. To analyze the impact of people's perceptions of luck on their support for economic relief, we should focus on luck in the context of the pandemic. This is because economic relief during the pandemic is most justified when one is suffering from bad luck related to the pandemic.

[COVID_economy_luck] Respondents read the following prompt: "Regarding the damage caused by COVID-19, there are two contrasting views, A and B. With which of the views do you agree? If anyone's employment or income is negatively influenced by the new coronavirus pandemic, I think it is due to …" Then, they choose from "1 A his or her self-responsibility," "2 close to A," "3 Neither A nor B," "4 close to B," and "5 B his or her bad luck."

The following analyses include several control variables. The first is people's anxiety about COVID-19 (Jørgensen et al., 2021; Rees-Jones et al., 2022). It is expected that people who are concerned about COVID-19 will be more likely (than those who are not concerned) to demand that the government take certain measures. In fact, studies have shown that people who are concerned about COVID-19 tend to support increased unemployment insurance and healthcare spending (Rees-Jones et al., 2022) and to positively evaluate COVID-19 control measures in general (Jørgensen et al., 2021). Thus, we include a variable based on the following item: "How likely is it that you think the following situation will happen? Within one year, you will be infected with coronavirus disease 2019 (COVID-19) and hospitalized. Please answer an approximate number."

We also include a variable to indicate whether the respondent suffered from a decrease in income after the pandemic began when analyzing determinants of people's support for economic relief during the pandemic. The experience of such economic loss leads one to seek economic support from the government. Accordingly, respondents who faced an income decrease after the pandemic began should be more likely to show a positive attitude toward economic support than those who did not.[5]

In addition, we include sociodemographic variables such as age, gender, and educational background, which Weisstanner (2022), for instance, found to impact people's preference for UBI. We also analyze the effects of subjective social class and political ideology (left or right).

The last control variable is support for the ruling party. There is consensus among existing studies that support for the ruling party determines people's approval of COVID-19 measures. Those who support the ruling party are more likely than those who do not to positively evaluate the government's overall COVID-19 measures (Jørgensen et al., 2021) and to positively evaluate both the government's policies to protect people's health and its economic measures (Altiparmakis et al., 2021). Analyzing data from several European countries, Jørgensen et al. (2021) reported that support for the ruling party had a positive effect, whereas support for either the left or right party had no effect. These findings suggest that the evaluation of COVID-19 policies depends more on whether the party one supports the policy than on whether the policy is close to one's own policy orientation. Yamamoto and Fujita (2023) confirmed this variable's influence in the context of Japan. This variable is used in the data analyses for Japan and Korea, which are democracies.

Results

Before moving to the multiple regression analysis, let us check the distribution of the responses of the dependent variables. Figure 7.3 shows the ratios of people's responses to the question item regarding orthodox redistribution policies. The ratio of agreement with the orthodox redistribution policy differs across China, Korea, and Japan. Seventy percent of the Chinese respondents, 57% of the Korean respondents, and 44% of the Japanese respondents reported positive attitudes toward orthodox redistribution policies. Negative attitudes toward such policies are less common among these countries, as fewer than 20% of respondents show negative attitudes.

Figure 7.4 shows the ratios of people's responses to the question regarding economic relief payments for individuals during the pandemic. As is the case for the ratio of support for orthodox redistribution, Japan, Korea, and China show, in that order, increasingly positive attitudes toward economic relief. Approximately 70% of the Chinese respondents, 40% of the Korean respondents, and 20% of the Japanese respondents responded positively to the economic relief during the pandemic. In the case of Japan, the portion of negative responses to economic relief is larger than that of positive responses. Do differences among countries in the perception of luck influence this pattern? The following statistical analysis at the individual level reveals whether this is the case.

Table 7.1 shows the results of an ordinal logistic regression analysis of East Asian countries' respondents, where the dependent variable is support for orthodox redistribution policies. The upper number of each cell indicates an odds ratio. The

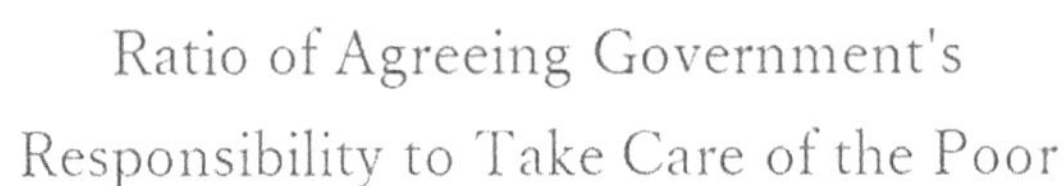

China (N = 1000) 2% 9% 20% 54% 16%
Korea (N = 1000) 4% 12% 27% 41% 16%
Japan (N = 1000) 3% 11% 41% 32% 12%
0% 20% 40% 60% 80% 100%
Strongly disagree
Disagree
Neither
Agree
Strongly agree

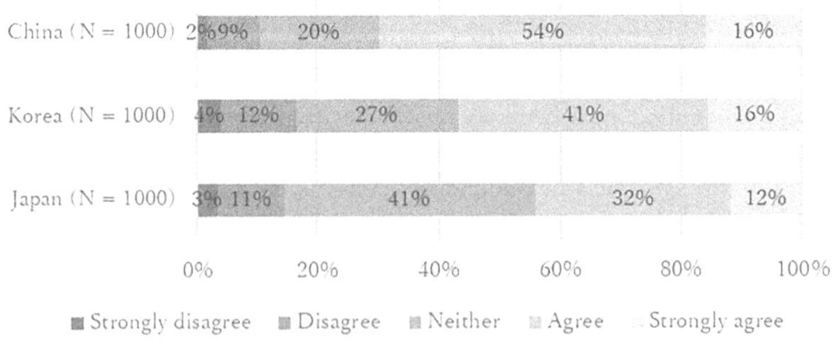

Figure 7.3 The ratio of approval of the government's measures to take care of those living in poverty.

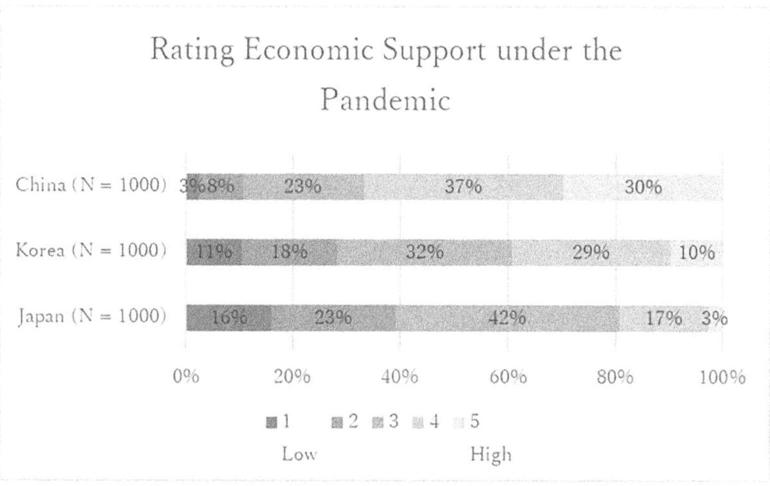

Figure 7.4 Support for economic relief payments during the pandemic.

Table 7.1 Ordinal logistic analysis of people's support for the orthodox redistribution policy in East Asian countries

	Japan	*South Korea*	*China*
Age	1.02*** (1.01–1.03)	1.01*** (1.00–1.02)	1.02*** (1.01–1.03)
Female	0.83 (0.64–1.07)	0.83 (0.65–1.04)	0.90 (0.69–1.17)
Class	1.03 (0.89–1.20)	0.98 (0.86–1.12)	1.17** (1.01–1.36)
Infection	1.00 (1.00–1.01)	1.00 (0.99–1.00)	0.95* (0.91–1.00)
Conservative	0.85*** (0.76–0.95)	0.95 (0.87–1.05)	0.82** (0.77–0.87)
Education	1.07 (0.81–1.40)	0.87 (0.68–1.10)	1.65** (1.22–2.24)
RULING_Party	1.22 (0.88–1.68)	1.20 (0.90–1.60)	
POOR_luck	1.66*** (1.43–1.92)	1.21*** (1.08–1.36)	0.98*** (1.22–2.24)
Observations	813	958	1000

Note: The table presents the odds ratios and lower and upper confidence limit (in parentheses) from the ordinal logistic regression.
* $p < .10$, ** $p < .05$, *** $p < .01$.

Table 7.2 Ordinal logistic analysis of people's support for economic relief payments during the pandemic in East Asian countries

	Japan	*South Korea*	*China*
AGE	1.00 (0.99–1.01)	1.01** (1.00–1.02)	1.00 (0.99–1.01)
Female	1.32** (1.02–1.71)	0.93 (0.74–1.18)	1.40*** (1.09–1.80)
Class	0.91 (0.78–1.06)	0.76*** (0.67–0.87)	0.89* (0.77–1.02)
Infection	1.00 (0.99–1.01)	1.00 (1.00–1.01)	0.96* (0.91–1.00)
Conservative	0.96 (0.86–1.07)	0.82*** (0.75–0.91)	0.88*** (0.83–0.94)
Education	0.88 (0.67–1.15)	0.77** (0.61–0.97)	0.90 (0.67–1.20)
RULING_Party	2.90*** (2.08–4.03)	1.38** (1.04–1.84)	
POOR_luck	1.00 (0.87–1.15)	1.24*** (1.11–1.38)	1.00 (0.89–1.13)
COVIDeconomy_luck	0.79*** (0.68–0.92)	0.88** (0.79–0.99)	0.88** (0.80–0.97)
COVID_INCOMEdecrease	0.65*** (0.55–0.78)	0.84*** (0.74–0.95)	0.87** (0.78–0.97)
Observations	813	958	1000

Note: The table presents the odds ratios and lower and upper confidence limit (in parentheses) from the ordinal logistic regression.
* $p < .10$, ** $p < .05$, *** $p < .01$.

odds ratio is a measure of the association between a cause and an outcome. It represents the odds that the level of an outcome will rise given a particular cause compared with the odds of the outcome occurring given a lower level of the cause. If the odds ratio of a cause is greater than 1.0, the cause positively influences the level of an outcome. In contrast, if the odds ratio of a cause is lower than 1.0, the cause negatively influences the level of an outcome.

The left column of Table 7.1 shows the analysis results for Japanese respondents. Respondents who consider being poor to be due to bad luck are more likely to show a positive response toward orthodox redistribution. This follows the pattern observed in Western countries by existing studies. Additionally, as expected, older respondents and those who are liberal are more likely to approve of orthodox redistribution. In contrast, gender, subjective social class, worry about infection by COVID-19, support for the ruling political party, and educational background did not have statistically significant effects. The finding that worries about infection do not have an influence might imply that the pandemic has not changed people's attitudes toward the orthodox redistribution policy in Japan. Even when we exclude the variable of support for the ruling party in line with the analysis of China, the results do not change in terms of which variable is statistically significant in which direction.

The middle column of Table 7.1 shows the results of an ordinal logistic regression analysis of Korean respondents, where the dependent variable is support for the orthodox redistribution policy. Like respondents in Japan, those who consider being poor due to bad luck are more likely to show a positive attitude toward orthodox redistribution policies. As expected, elderly and male respondents are more likely to approve of orthodox redistribution. In contrast, other variables, including ideology, do not have a statistically significant effect. Excluding the variable of support for the ruling party does not change the results.

The right column of Table 7.1 shows the results of an ordinal logistic regression analysis of Chinese respondents, where the dependent variable is support for orthodox redistribution policies. Unlike in Japan or Korea, whether a respondent considers being poor to result from bad luck is not a determinant of whether that respondent shows a positive attitude toward the orthodox redistribution policy. As expected, age and liberal ideology make respondents likely to approve of orthodox redistribution. In contrast, high subjective social class and high educational background positively affect support for orthodox redistribution, which is contrary to our expectations.

Table 7.2 shows the results of an ordinal logistic regression analysis, whose dependent variable is support for economic relief payments during the pandemic. The left column of Table 7.2 shows the analysis results for Japanese respondents. Surprisingly, respondents who consider individual economic damage triggered by the pandemic to be due to bad luck are less likely to show a positive attitude toward economic relief during the pandemic.

The experience of economic damage due to the pandemic also decreases support for economic relief. Again, the result is opposite to our expectations. Control variables other than gender and support for the ruling party are not determinants, contrary to what we expected on the basis of existing studies and conventional understanding. Age, social class, concern about COVID-19 infection, ideology, and educational background did not have statistically significant effects. Female and the support of the ruling party has a positive effect on support for economic relief, which follows existing studies' findings that people evaluate COVID-19 countermeasures according not to the content of the measure but to the political position of the decision maker.[6] Even the perception that being poor is due to bad luck does not influence support for economic relief during the pandemic.

Thus, there are clearly many differences in the determinants of Japanese people's support for orthodox redistribution policies and economic relief during the pandemic.

The middle column of Table 7.2 shows the results of an ordinal logistic regression analysis of Korean respondents, where the dependent variable is support for economic relief payments during the pandemic. Like respondents in Japan, those who consider individual negative impacts on individuals' economic circumstances triggered by the pandemic to be due to bad luck are less likely to show a positive posture toward economic relief during the pandemic, although this is not at the 5% significance level (rather at the 10% level).

The experience of economic damage due to the pandemic also decreases support for economic relief. The results in Korea are the opposite of our expectations as well. In contrast to Japan, many control variables, such as age, subjective social class, ideological position, and educational background, influence support for economic relief during the pandemic. The control variables, except for gender and concern about infection, have a statistically significant effect in the expected direction. Support for the ruling party has a positive effect on support for economic relief, which follows the findings of existing studies.[7] Unlike in Japan, the perception that being poor is due to bad luck influences support for economic relief during the pandemic, as it does support orthodox redistribution in Korea.

In summary, first, bad luck in the context of the pandemic seems not to be a reason to support economic relief among Koreans. Second, however, the determinants of support for economic relief are similar to those of support for orthodox redistribution. Koreans and Japanese are similar in terms of the first point but not the second.

The right column of Table 7.2 shows the results of an ordinal logistic regression analysis of Chinese respondents, where the dependent variable is support for economic relief payments during the pandemic. Like respondents in Japan and Korea, those who consider negative impacts on individuals' economic situation triggered by the pandemic to be due to bad luck are less likely to show a positive attitude toward economic relief during the pandemic, although not at the 5% significance level (rather at the 10% level).

Those in China who suffer negative economic impacts from the pandemic are also less likely to support economic relief, as are those in Japan and Korea. The results in China also contradict our expectations. The control variables of gender and ideology have the expected impacts on support for economic relief during the pandemic. Women and liberal respondents tend to support economic relief. Those worried about infection by COVID-19 are less likely to support relief, contrary to our expectation, though not at a statistically significant level (rather at the 10% level). The other control variables do not have a statistically significant influence.

In short, bad luck in the context of the pandemic does not seem to be a strong reason for Chinese people to support economic relief as it was not for Japanese and Korean people.

Discussion and Conclusion

This chapter aims to answer two research questions. The first research question concerns whether people's thoughts about the role of luck determine their support for economic relief payments during the pandemic as well as their support for orthodox redistribution policies. On the one hand, the analyses in this chapter show that people's belief that luck determines one's outcomes leads people to support orthodox redistribution in Japan and Korea but not in China. On the other hand, respondents who thought that the negative economic impacts of COVID-19 resulted from bad luck were more likely to disapprove of the state's economic support during the pandemic, which was similar across the three countries. Thus, we observed a clear contrast in the effect of luck between orthodox redistribution and economic relief during the pandemic, at least in Japan and Korea. People seem to consider that the aim of COVID-19 economic relief is not to solve the impact of luck. People do not seem to believe that inequality due to bad luck during the COVID-19 pandemic should be minimized. The state's economic role during the pandemic is perceived to be different from that of the orthodox redistribution policy.[8] Considering that the proportion of those supporting economic relief during the pandemic was lower than that for orthodox redistribution policies at the national level across the three countries, we can conclude that people in East Asian countries are unlikely to approve of UBI. This result implies that COVID-19 has not made people expect the expansion of the state's economic role.

The second research question in this chapter concerns whether there is a difference between East Asian countries in the influence of people's thoughts about luck on their support for the state's economic role. The analysis of multidimensional patterns in people's perceptions of luck revealed that Korean respondents consistently believe that luck plays a notable role in many different contexts, unlike Japanese and Chinese respondents. This difference seems to explain the difference in the determinants of support for economic relief during the pandemic. Although bad luck in the context of the pandemic has a negative impact on support for economic relief payments in Korea, Korean respondents who attribute being poor to bad luck are more likely to show positive attitudes toward economic relief payments. Moreover, among Korean respondents, the variables that cause individuals to support orthodox redistribution, such as age, subjective social class, ideological position, and educational background, also lead individuals to support economic relief during the pandemic. Hence, we can conclude that of the three East Asian countries, the Korean people are distinctive in that they hold a somewhat Rawlsian perspective and view economic relief during the pandemic.

This chapter's analyses cannot explain why only Koreans but not Japanese and Chinese people hold a Rawlsian perspective. Nevertheless, it is evident that factors such as the political regime, welfare regime, and average living standard are not determinants of the difference, because such factors do not differ between Korea and Japan.

The effect of the perception of the role of luck may differ in Western countries, where the damage caused by COVID-19 has been much greater than that in East Asian countries. Likewise, it could be that people in East Asian countries changed their thinking after the negative effects of COVID-19 increased toward the end of 2022. Nevertheless, it is critical to show how East Asian residents thought about the state's economic role as of the beginning of 2022. Our findings enable us to measure changes before and after the surge in the negative effects of COVID-19.

Acknowledgment

This research was supported by the Japan Society for the Promotion of Science (JSPS) Grants-in-Aid for Scientific Research [grant number 20H00061]; Murata Scientific Foundation; the Nagasaki University State of the Art Research program.

Notes

1 Studies have empirically shown that inherent luck, such as a month of birth, affects career success (e.g., Du et al., 2012; Muller and Page, 2016; Yamaguchi et al., 2023). Koizumi (2024) persuasively shows that even if people are equal in terms of talent and family background, luck on merit in the absence of initial differences in individual characteristics has a significant impact on one's achievement. That is, the fairness of meritocracy is doubtful, as luck plays a role, even under meritocracy.

2 There are some variants of arguments on just society that emphasize the role of luck in inequality. For example, "luck egalitarians" such as Dworkin (2000) consider the distinction between the result of luck and that of choice critical, and only the former is unjust. In contrast, scholars such as Persson (2006) argue that talent, effort, and even choice are determined by luck. Regardless of the difference in the range of impact that luck has on inequality, the point here is that luck's role has been considered critical. Rawls is the most prominent scholar who pioneered the argument based on luck.

3 In China, the target of the government's economic support (giving cash) for individuals and households has not been all the citizens but has been limited to those living in poverty.

4 Macchia and Ariely (2021) found that people have different preferences across domains. They accept higher inequality in wealth whereas they prefer more equal distributions in education and health.

5 The wording of the question item for this variable is "What did you think about the situation around you after the coronavirus pandemic began?" The response choices are a little different among countries. In China, after reading "I and/or any of my family experienced the decrease in income due to the coronavirus (Covid-19) pandemic," respondents choose from "1 not at all" to "5 very much." In Japan and Korea, respondents read "After the pandemic began, your income and your household's income …" and choose from "1 A increased," "2 close to A," "3 Neither A nor B," "4 close to B," "5 B decreased."

6 Excluding the variable of the support for government party in line with the analysis of China does not change the results.

7 Excluding the variable of the support for government party in line with the analysis of China does not change the results.

8 One might think that a reason for the contrast lies in the difference in the content of payment between the two distribution policies: while all individuals receive the same amount for economic relief payments during the pandemic, the orthodox redistribution method pay different amounts depending on the recipient's economic situation. Considering even respondents who believe in luck are less likely to support economic relief even in China where payments of the same amount have not been paid to all individuals, this seems to not be the case.

References

Alesina, Alberto F, Edward Glaeser, and Bruce Sacerdote. 2001. Why doesn't the United States have a European-style welfare state? *Brookings Papers on Economic Activity* 2001(2): 187–254.

Altiparmakis, Argyrios, Abel Bojar, Sylvain Brouard, Martial Foucault, Hanspeter Kriesi, and Richard Nadeau. 2021. Pandemic politics: Policy evaluations of government responses to Covid-19. *West European Politics* 44(5–6): 1159–1179.

Ares, Macarena, Reto Bürgisser, and Silja Häusermann. 2021. Attitudinal polarization towards the redistributive role of the state in the wake of the Covid-19 crisis. *Journal of Elections, Public Opinion and Parties* 31(1): 41–55.

Bénabou, Roland, and Jean Tirole. 2016. Mindful economics: The production, consumption, and value of beliefs. *Journal of Economic Perspectives* 30(3): 141–164.

Blumenau, Jack, Timothy Hicks, Alan Jacobs, Scott Matthews, and Tom O'Grady. 2021. Testing negative: The non-consequences of COVID-19 on mass ideology. American Political Science Association Preprints, September 29, 2021. https://preprints.apsanet.org/engage/apsa/article-details/61530c5fd1fc334936f71953

Daniele, Gianmarco, Andrea Martinangeli, Francesco Passarelli, Willem Sas, and Lisa Windsteiger. 2020. Wind of change? Experimental survey evidence on the Covid-19 shock and socio-political attitudes in Europe. *CESifo Working Paper* No. 8517.

Du, Qianqian, Huasheng Gao, Maurice D. Levi. 2012. The relative-age effect and career success: Evidence from corporate CEOs. *Economics Letters* 117(3): 660–662.

Dworkin, Ronald. 2000. *Sovereign Virtue*. Cambridge MA: Harvard University Press.

Engelmann, Dirk, and Martin Strobel. 2004. Inequality aversion, efficiency, and maximin preferences in simple distribution experiments. *American Economic Review* 94(4): 857–869.

Fong, Christina. 2001. Social preferences, self-interest, and the demand for redistribution. *Journal of Public Economics* 82(2): 225–246.

Frohlich, Norman and Joe A. Oppenheimer. 1992. *Choosing Justice: An Experimental Approach to Ethical Theory*. Berkeley: University of California Press.

Jørgensen, Frederik, Alexander Bor, Marie Fly Lindholt, and Michael Bang Petersen. 2021. Public support for government responses against Covid-19: Assessing levels and predictors in eight western democracies during 2020. *West European Politics* 44(5–6): 1129–1158.

Kameda, Tatsuya, Keigo Inukai, Satomi Higuchi, Akitoshi Ogawa, Hackjin Kim, Tetsuya Matsuda, and Masamichi Sakagami. 2016. Rawlsian maximin rule operates as a common cognitive anchor in distributive justice and risky decisions. *Proceedings of the National Academy of Sciences* 113(42): 11817–11822.

Klemm, Alexander, and Paolo Mauro. 2022. Pandemic and progressivity. *International Tax and Public Finance* 29(2): 505–535.

Koizumi, Hideto. 2024. How Much of Merit Is Due to Luck? Evidence on the Butterfly Effect of Luck. *RIETI Discussion Paper Series* 24-E-035 March 2024.

Macchia, Lucia and Dan Ariely. 2021. Eliciting preferences for redistribution across domains: A study on wealth, education, and health. *Analyses of Social Issues and Public Policy* 21(1): 1141–1166.

Muller, Daniel, Lionel Page, Born Leaders. 2016. Political selection and the relative age effect in the US congress. *Journal of the Royal Statistical Society Series A: Statistics in Society* 179(3): 809–829.

Nettle, Daniel, Elliott Johnson, Matthew Johnson, and Rebecca Saxe. 2021. Why has the COVID-19 pandemic increased support for universal basic income? *Humanities and Social Sciences Communications* 8: 79.

Norton, Michael I, and Dan Ariely. 2011. Building a better America—One wealth quintile at a time. *Perspectives on Psychological Science* 6(1): 9–12.

Osberg, Lars, and Timothy Smeeding. 2006. "Fair" inequality? Attitudes toward pay differentials: The United States in comparative perspective. *American Sociological Review* 71(3): 450–473.

Persson, Ingmar. 2006. A defence of extreme egalitarianism. In Nils Holtug and Kasper Lippert-Rasmussen (eds.), *Egalitarianism: New Essays on the Nature and Value of Equality*. Oxford: Oxford University Press, pp. 83–98.

Rawls, John. 1971. *A Theory of Justice*. Cambridge, MA: Belknap Press of Harvard University Press.

Rees-Jones, Alex, John D'Attoma, Amedeo Piolatto, and Luca Salvadori. 2022. Experience of the Covid-19 pandemic and support for safety-net expansion. *Journal of Economic Behavior & Organization* 200: 1090–1104.

Reeskens, Tim, Quita Muis, Inge Sieben, Leen Vandecasteele, Ruud Luijkx, and Loek Halman. 2021. Stability or change of public opinion and values during the Coronavirus crisis? Exploring Dutch longitudinal panel data. *European Societies* 23(1): S153–S171.

Sandel, Michael J. 2007. *The Case against Perfection: Ethics in the Age of Genetic Engineering*. Cambridge: Harvard University Press.

Sandel, Michael J. 2020. *The Tyranny of Merit: What's Become of the Common Good?* London: Penguin Press.

Van Parijs, Philippe. 2004. Basic income: A simple and powerful idea for the twenty-first century. *Politics & Society* 32(1): 7–39.

Weisstanner, David. 2022. COVID-19 and welfare state support: The case of universal basic income. *Policy and Society* 41(1): 96–110.

Yamaguchi, Shintaro, Hirotake Ito, Makiko Nakamuro. 2023. Month-of-birth Effects on Skills and Skill formation. *Labour Economics* 84: 102392.

Yamamoto, Hidehiro, and Taisuke Fujita. 2023. State-society relations under the COVID disaster in Japan. In Jozef Oleński, Jeffrey Sachs, Masayuki Susai, Yannis Tsekouras, and Arjan Gjonça (eds.), *Handbook of Research on Socio-Economic Sustainability in the Post-Pandemic Era*. Hershey: IGI Global, pp. 139–157.

Part III

Beyond the National Boundaries

8 A Comparative Study of the Citizen Assessments of COVID-19 Governance in Japan, South Korea, and China

Sang-Jin Han

Data and Methodologies

In this investigation, two primary sources of data were employed. One is an online global survey on "COVID-19 and Civic Life" that was carried out in September 2021 by the Joongmin Foundation in Korea,[1] targeting citizens from 33 major cities, under a contract with Rakuten, a Japanese firm that specializes in conducting international survey researches. The survey format was a questionnaire. Despite the wide scope of its survey items, this chapter utilizes only one item relating to the evaluations of citizens from 33 global cities about COVID-19 quarantine performance, with a special emphasis on the governments of Japan, South Korea, and China.

The other data set, and the most important data set for this study, comes from an online poll that the present book's editors performed in 2022 with a sample of 1,000 citizens each from China, Korea, and Japan. Since all of the chapters in this book made use of this data which is referred to as the "EASA RN IPS Joint Research Survey," an explanation of the survey including the sample's demographics, is not included in this chapter.

A crucial methodological question for this chapter is how to compare the COVID-19 governance of Japan, South Korea, and China and within what conceptual framework. The chapter is innovative in that it attempts to construct four conceptual types of COVID-19 governance rather than pursuing a descriptive comparison of each question asked. For this, using the EASA RN IPS Joint Research Survey, this chapter identifies the key variables and axes by which governance types can be constructed and shows the defining characteristics and variations of each governance type, as well as their distribution and impacts by country. Furthermore, an attempt was made to measure ten (10) indices of the COVID-19 quarantine system. The impacts of the four types of governance were analyzed based on these efforts.

DOI: 10.4324/9781003495239-11

A Striking Tendency in the East Asian Assessments of COVID-19 Governance

Considerable researches have been carried out to investigate the distinctive characteristics of COVID-19 experience and quarantine policies in the world, including Japan, South Korea, and China (Boeing and Wang, 2021; Degerman, 2020; Domingues, 2022; Q. Han, 2020; S. Han, 2020a, 2020b, 2020c, 2023; He et al., 2020; Hosoda, 2023; Jing, 2021; Prasad, 2022; Rolland, 2020; Shim, 2023; Wang, 2022). Seldom, however, a comparative study in the rigorous sense has been conducted, perhaps due to the policy of the Chinese government to repress international comparative survey research and discourse on COVID-19 within mainland of China. Yet today it is possible to pursue this, and this chapter is an example.

Before diving into an analytical comparative analysis of the three East Asian countries of Japan, South Korea, and China, I first want to take a quick look at the features of the citizen assessments coming out of East Asia from a global standpoint. The fascinating thing is that the perceptions of "East Asia" among East Asians differed significantly from those of global citizens. People who live in Japan, South Korea, and China—three countries with long independent histories and close geographic proximity—view one another with extremely sensitive and picky attitudes. They compete fiercely with one another. They do not hide their ethnocentric tendencies when evaluating their neighbors. Strong pride leads to stingy evaluations with respect to others. This can be confirmed with regard to COVID-19 quarantine. It is evident that people around the world hold a very positive evaluation of Korea, Japan, China, and East Asia as a whole. The quarantine systems in East Asia were thought to be the best in the world. The three East Asian countries do not, however, cheer one another on. They readily point out each other's shortcomings while being stingy in acknowledging each other's strengths. The intense rivalry among the three countries, as well as their deep-rooted tension over problems of history, appear to have blocked a mutually respecting communication and opened a profound psychological divide among them.

I will briefly examine the data from the "COVID-19 and Civic Life" survey conducted in September 2021. The data was drawn from 500 samples chosen at random from 33 global cities, based on age (all 19 years of age or older) and gender. Collecting a total of 17,564 global samples in this way, a web survey was conducted from August 18 to September 16, 2021, to uncover the particularities of the assessments made by citizens from East Asia. This analysis served as the background and the starting point of the present research.[2]

More specifically, the survey item used in this chapter dealt with the assessment of national health performance: "Please evaluate how competent the governments of the following countries have been in dealing with the COVID-19 pandemic," together with a list of 33 countries plus China (PRC). A 5-point scale (1–5) was given ranging from "Very Competent" to "Very Incompetent" including N/A. This means that global citizens could evaluate the COVID-19 performance of the mainland Chinese government even though no mainland Chinese city was included in the survey due to strict policy by the People's Republic of China.

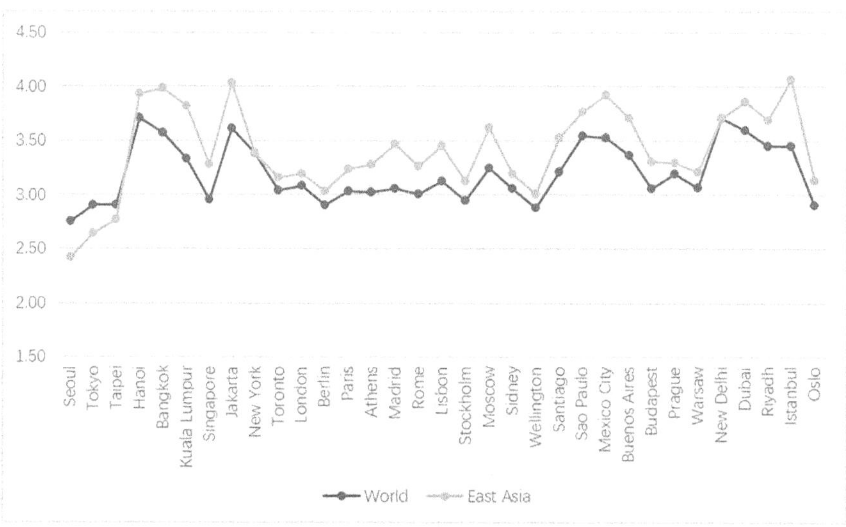

Figure 8.1 Comparison of the average assessments of East Asia by global and East Asian citizens. Please stretch the figure 8.1 to the right direction maching with the title of the figure.

Figure 8.1 demonstrates how citizens in each of the 33 cities felt about the performance of COVID-19 governance across the globe at two levels. The first is related to what we may call "global performance" and the second "East Asian" performance. Figure 8.1 compares the global average score and the East Asian average score by city. For example, in the case of Seoul, the global average score is higher than the East Asian average score. This means that the citizens of Seoul see East Asian performance of COVID-19 governance including Japan, South Korea, and China to be lagging behind the global average score collected from the 33 cities under survey. A similar tendency can be confirmed in the cases of Tokyo and Taipei. This tendency contrasts strikingly with the patterns observed in all other cities, as exemplified by the gap between the two types of average scores.

To reiterate a bit further, in Figure 8.1, "World" represents the global average of scores by city. The higher the average, the better the COVID-19 governance. On the other hand, "East Asia" represents the East Asian average of scores by city. The latter shows how the citizens of 33 global cities evaluate the performance of East Asian countries, that is, Japan, South Korea, and China. As illustrated in Figure 8.1, the criteria for assessment vary from city to city. For instance, the citizens from Hanoi, Jakarta, and New Delhi show the highest global average score. However, East Asia is exactly the opposite. The data analysis shows that every single city outside of Seoul, Tokyo, and Taipei rated East Asian COVID-19 performance significantly and consistently higher than their global average scores. That is, the global perception of 33 cities of East Asian COVID-19 performance was far higher than their global perception of the COVID-19 governance in all other countries under survey. This methodology of comparing the average scores by city for "East Asia" with those for "World" is deemed to be trustworthy.[3]

What deserves attention is the fact that the East Asian average scores collected from East Asian citizens consistently fell short of their global average. This indicates that, in their opinion, the performances of COVID-19 governance in Japan, South Korea, and Japan were noticeably below the estimated worldwide average. The gap between "World" and "East Asia" was not so great for Taipei citizens, but it was significant for Seoul and Tokyo citizens.

Nevertheless, notable disparities arise when comparing East Asian assessments of COVID-19 governance in China, Korea, and Japan. The Seoul citizens appeared to think that Korea performed significantly better than China or Japan. Overall, they saw China, Japan, and Korea as having vastly different performance levels from each other in terms of COVID-19 governance. Tokyo citizens saw COVID-19 governance in China and Japan as essentially the same but thought Korea's performance was better than theirs. Taipei respondents believed that Korea performed well, followed by Japan, and saw China as underdeveloped.

The country whose scores for COVID-19 governance differed greatest between "World" and "East Asia" was Japan. People outside of East Asia believed that Japan's COVID-19 governance was far superior to the global average. In Kuala Lumpur, New York, Toronto, Berlin, and New Delhi, the difference between the average for "World" and for Japan was not as great, but in other places the difference was conspicuous. That is, Japan's performance during the COVID-19 quarantine was well regarded globally. But once in East Asia, things take a different turn. Japan's performance is rated marginally below the global average by Taipei citizens, and significantly below the global average for Seoul citizens. Even in the case of Tokyo citizens Japan's performance turned out to be well below the global average.

Within East Asia, assessments of Korea's success were also contentious. Seoul citizens gave Korea an average score that was much higher than their global average. However, Tokyo citizens perceived Korea's performance as lower than their global average, while Taipei citizens perceived it as somewhat better. On the other hand, people living outside of East Asia, in every city but Athens, believed that Korea performed really well.

These findings indicate a significant discrepancy with respect to the performance of COVID-19 governance between East Asian and global assessments. This demonstrates how competitive, overcritical, and sensitive East Asians may be toward one another, which can occasionally become a source of friction and strife.

Four Conceptual Models for COVID-19 Governance

Construction of the Four Models

The starting point of this comparative approach is to formulate the various types of COVID-19 governance and use the survey data referred to as the EASA RN IPS

Joint Research Survey to analyze each type's scope and distribution by country. As a result of the COVID-19 crisis, robust national systems and several emergency protocols were implemented globally. However, there are two pressing public issues from the perspective of citizens. Should one favor a national system that sacrifices individual freedom for the purposes of quarantine and disease eradication such as limits on population movement, immigration control, and social distancing campaigns? Or should one favor the rule of law, even when it comes to public health, carrying out measures in a way that upholds individual freedom? This is a matter of value judgment, and the answer will determine the fundamental structure of the order that the public supports. The second issue relates to the proper agency of quarantine. To simplify the issue, a choice must be made between viewing the government as the main agency of quarantine and emphasizing the government's responsibility, or viewing the subject of quarantine as the individual and emphasizing the individual's role in responding to the COVID-19 issue. The answer will determine the central agency in charge of quarantine.

Depending on the first choice, different trends may emerge ranging from the liberal tradition that prioritizes personal autonomy and decision-making, to emphasis on the rule of law. In terms of the latter choice, other different tendencies can be identified, ranging from a state of "exception" that upholds order while tolerating strict measures such as emergency orders, to communitarianism that balances individual rights and the good of the community.

Drawing from this theoretical explanatory scheme, the following questions were used in this research as constituent factors of the COVID-19 governance types.

Regarding the measures against COVID-19, there are two contrasting views, A and B. With which of the views do you agree? Please use this scale to indicate your position.

A. The restriction of liberty is inevitable to prevent the spread of infections.			Middle	B. The restriction of liberty is not desirable even if the purpose is to prevent the spread of infections.		
1	2	3	4	5	6	7

A. It is the individual's responsibility to prevent infection.			middle	B. It is the government's responsibility to prevent infection.		
1	2	3	4	5	6	7

Simple frequencies for the two components were generated, as follows: The responses were arranged on a 7-point scale, making it impossible to identify the middle point on the scale corresponding to the "order model" that citizens prefer. Therefore, for convenience, all responses in the 1–3 point range were combined, yielding a percentage of 66% classified as "preference for regulation"; and all responses in the 4–7 point range were combined, yielding a percentage of 44% classified as "preference for freedom." With respect to the agency of quarantine, scores ranging from 1 to 3 (48.9% of the responses) were classified as "individual-centered," and scores ranging from 4 to 7 (51.1% of the responses) as "government-centered." Concerning the preferred model of order, one may insist that scores in the 1–2 point range (45.1%) can be classified as "preference for regulation." However, on the given 7-point scale, putting the dividing line at three makes greater sense.

As seen in Table 8.1, the two axes forming the COVID-19 governance model were intersected to produce four models.

The four types of governance thus distinguished refer to the preferred types of order by East Asian citizens, not to any objective reality in East Asian politics. The "Liberal Democratic State," which makes up the smallest percentage (10.1%) in East Asia, is distinguished by its politico-philosophical emphasis on individual freedom and personal accountability in connection to the COVID-19 quarantine. Those who want this form of government frequently hold the view that each person bears responsibility for their own health-related issues, including COVID-19 infection. The defense of both the principle of individual freedom and the active role of the government can be described as the "Rule of Law Intervention State." The 23.9% of East Asian citizens who supported this form of government feel that, in times of emergency like the COVID-19 pandemic, the state should defend individual rights by upholding the rule of law while strengthening its capability in socioeconomic intervention. The hallmark of the "Communitarian Regulative State," which is home to 38.9% of East Asian citizens, is its emphasis on the function of a sustainable community while upholding an individual's role as a quarantine agent (Hillenbrand, 2010). These supporters think that government policies should be based on the cooperation of individuals. They also consider the responsibilities undertaken by regions, workplaces, churches, interest groups, residential communities, and so on. They find particularly ideal a form of welfare administration in which people actively work together to ensure that the weak can coexist with the strong. Last but not least, the term "Rule by Order Exceptional State" describes the kind of strong

Table 8.1 Governance types

		Preferred order		
		Liberal	Regulative	Total
Actor	Individual role	Liberal Democratic State	Communitarian Regulative State	48.9% (1,468)
	Individual role (cut)	10.1% (302)	38.9% (1,166)	48.9% (1,468)
	Government role	Rule of Law Intervention State	Rule by Order Exceptional State	51.1% (1,532)
	Government role (cut)	23.9% (718)	27.1% (814)	51.1% (1,532)
	Total	34.0% (1,020)	66.0% (1,980)	100.0% (3,000)

authoritarian state that Agamben (2005) and Schmitt (1934) supported. It is a style of government that emerges from a crisis when the nation's existence is threatened, by implementing drastic emergency measures, including the use of extralegal means.

Types of Governance by Nationality

The distribution of the four governance types in each East Asian country turned out as follows with the chi-square test, 51.946 ($p = .000$). Overall, 10.1% of East Asian citizens favored a Liberal Democratic State, with Korea making up the highest percentage. About 23.9% of East Asian citizens favor a Rule of Law Intervention State, split evenly among China, Japan, and Korea, with Korea again making up the highest percentage. This could indicate that, out of all citizens in East Asia, Koreans place the highest importance on freedom. However, 38.9% of East Asian citizens, particularly those in Japan, formed the majority that favored a Communitarian Regulative State. Last but not least, the Rule by Order Exceptional State—which is particularly prevalent in China—is preferred by 27.1% of East Asians. This administration type was preferred by citizens of China (31.2%) and Korea (28.8%); in Japan, the percentage was only 21.4%.

By country, a greater percentage of people in Japan—44.8%—chose a Communitarian Regulative State than any other COVID-19 form of governance. This percentage was twice as high as the preferences for the Rule of Law Intervention State (23.4% of Japanese citizens) and the Exceptional State (21.4% of Japanese citizens). A similar distribution of preferences for the Rule of Law Intervention State, Communitarian Regulative State, and Rule by Order Exceptional State defined Korea. In contrast, the majority of Chinese citizens—38.9%—chose the Communitarian Regulative State, while a sizable portion—31.2%—chose the Rule by Order Exceptional State.

The most obvious tendency seen across East Asia was that a much higher proportion of people in China, Japan, and Korea favored a Communitarian Regulative State. This demonstrates the strong roots and impact of community-oriented culture and way of life established in East Asia.

The Ten Indices

Ten indices were developed to assess the efficiency of COVID-19 governance in the three East Asian countries. Every index has a connection to the state's involvement in the COVID-19 pandemic. The "general trust" and "political system efficiency" indices are not, strictly speaking, indices; rather, they are measured using a single question. Nonetheless, they are grouped with the others since they are primary factors that this study aimed to validate. The following is a description of how each index was constructed. Cronbach's alpha was used to gauge inter-item reliability, and Eigenvalues and factor loadings were provided by an exploratory factor analysis utilizing principal factor analysis.

Cause of COVID-19 Damage Index

The "cause of COVID-19 damage" index determined whether COVID-19-related damage was seen as the result of individual responsibility or "bad luck." To create the index, the average of a 5-point rating system was used to ascertain if personal or unlucky circumstances contributed to the "COVID-19 virus infection" and the "negative impact on employment or income due to COVID-19." The greater the index, the greater the perception of personal accountability for the harm inflicted by COVID-19. For the two questions, the Cronbach's alpha was 0.7546.

More specifically, the questions asked include "If anyone became infected with the new coronavirus, I think it was due to bad luck or one's lack of self-responsibility" and "If anyone's employment or income was negatively influenced by the new coronavirus, I think it was due to bad luck or one's lack of self-responsibility." Eigenvalue is 0.9791.

COVID-19 Entry Restrictions Index

The "COVID-19 entry restrictions" index, which consists of "foreigner entry restrictions" and "national citizen entry restrictions," was calculated based on the degree to which respondents agreed that entry limits should be put in place to stop the virus from spreading. It was computed as the mean of a 5-point scale, with higher values denoting agreement. The two questions' Cronbach's alpha was 0.7783.

More specifically, the questions asked include: "The government should restrict the entry of foreigners from abroad to contain the pandemic," and "The government should restrict the entry of Chinese/Korean/Japanese from abroad to contain the pandemic." Eigenvalue is 1.0428.

Government Support Index

The "government support" index was used to assess the government's economic assistance to companies, individuals, and households as a benchmark against COVID-19. Items rated with a larger figure denoted a higher quality; Cronbach's alpha was determined to be 0.7984.

More specifically, the questions asked include: "Government's economic support for businesses" and "Government's economic support for individuals and households." Eigenvalue is 1.1121.

Strengthening State Role Index

The "strengthening state role" index is made up of statements about the state's role with respect to the management of COVID-19 damage and was reverse-coded so that higher figures denoted agreement. Four questions were used to measure the results of an exploratory factor analysis that was based on an eigenvalue of 1 and a factor loading of 0.6. This question had a Cronbach alpha of 0.7860.

More specifically, the questions asked include the following four items:

"It is important for governments to provide more job and skills training for workers."
"The government should shrink income inequality more than they are doing now."
"The government should invest in promoting new industries such as green economy than they are doing now."
"The government should create jobs in new industries at the expense of old industries."

In this index, eigenvalue is 1.8116.

Nationalism Index

The "nationalism" index was generated using state-specific questions related to China, Japan, and Korea. Only questions with a factor loading of 0.6 or higher were included in the exploratory factor analysis employed to identify factors, and the average of the questions was calculated to create the index. Cronbach's alpha was 0.7760; the higher the figure, the more agreement there was with the concept.

More specifically, the questions asked include the following three items:

"Other countries should aspire to be like China/Korea/Japan."
"Generally, the more influence China/Korea/Japan has on other nations, the better off the latter are."
"It is important that China/Korea/Japan win in international sporting competitions like the Olympics."

In this index, eigenvalue is 1.4634.

Authoritarianism Index (Wish for a Strong Leader)

The "authoritarianism" index was measured using the "wish for a strong leader" index by Sprong et al. (2019). Three statements were used to elicit responses: (1) *Our country needs a strong leader right now*, (2) *We need strong leadership to ensure the society survives*, and (3) *We need strong leadership to overcome societies' difficulties.* Cronbach's alpha for all three statements was 0.9205, which is comparable to Sprong et al. (2019). The responses ranged from 1 (strongly disagree) to 7 (strongly agree).

Strict Emergency Protocols Index

The "strict emergency protocols" index was calculated based on the degree to which the respondent agreed with the following statements.

"In emergencies, it is better to follow government requests for restrictions on freedom of movement."
"In emergencies, it is better to follow government requests for restrictions on freedom of speech."
"In emergencies, anyone who goes out against government lockdown policy should be punished by law."
"In emergencies, speech contrary to government policy should be punished by law."

As usual, the higher the figure, the higher the support for the idea that immediate action is necessary.

The Cronbach's alpha and eigenvalue are 0.8157 and 2.0910, respectively.

Superiority of Democracy Index

The "superiority of democracy" index was calculated based on questions gauging the degree of agreement with statements about democracy and democratic nations. Positive descriptions of democracy were coded so that higher figures corresponded to higher levels of agreement; the resulting Cronbach's alpha was 0.8012.

More specifically, the questions asked include the following three items:

"Democracies are better political regimes than the others."
"Democratic countries have succeeded in managing the pandemic better than non-democratic countries."
"Democratic countries have succeeded in managing economic growth better than non-democratic countries."

In this index, eigenvalue is 1.5904.

General Trust Index

The "general trust" index has been employed by numerous studies as a measurement of overall societal trust. The question *Generally speaking, would you say you strongly agree, somewhat agree, somewhat disagree, or strongly disagree with the statement that "most people can be trusted"?* was used in China to assess the degree of agreement on a 5-point scale. The question asked in Korea and Japan was *In general, would you say that most people can be trusted or that you need to be very careful in dealing with people?* The higher the score, the more trust the respondent expressed. A 5-point rating system was also used to answer the question.

Political System Efficiency Index

The "political system efficiency" index was calculated by measuring responses to the statement "Our country's political system was prepared to deal efficiently with the pandemic." It was assessed using questionnaires and a 7-point grading system that went from 1 (strongly disagree) to 7 (strongly agree).

Findings

Comparison of Indices by Government Type

Table 8.2 shows the effects of the four COVID-19 governance models on the ten indices outlined above. For ease of reference, Table 8.2 designates the Rule of Law Intervention State as RIS, the Communitarian Regulative State as CRS, the Rule by Order Exceptional State as RES, and the Liberal Democratic State as LDS. To compare averages, one-way analysis of variance (ANOVA) was used, and Scheffe was used for the post hoc test.

An examination of the findings in Table 8.2 showed that there were statistically significant disparities in the impacts of governance types favored by East Asian citizens for the ten indices. Those who favored a Rule of Law Intervention State, in particular, showed distinct inclinations. Their stance is generally against entry restrictions, they oppose economic support from the government, they oppose a big government role, and they reject nationalistic and authoritarian tendencies.

Table 8.2 Index by governance type

	LDS	*RIS*	*CRS*	*RES*	*F (Scheffe)*
Cause of Covid-19 damage	4.939	4.716	4.664	4.846	14.069** (LDS>RIS=CRS, RES>CRS)
Entry restrictions	3.391	3.318	3.738	3.643	33.400*** (CRS=RES>LDS=RIS)
Government's support	3.119	2.891	3.443	3.298	135.213*** (CRS>RES>LDS>RIS)
Strengthening state role	3.728	3.603	3.929	4.038	56.750*** (RES>CRS>LDS=RIS)
Nationalism	5.082	4.896	5.405	5.241	45.990*** (CRS>RES=LDS>RIS)
Authoritarianism	5.407	5.047	5.686	5.620	45.380*** (CRS=RES>RIS, CRS>LDS>RIS)
Strict emergency Protocols	4.315	4.110	5.178	4.800	133.070*** (CRS>RES>LDS=RIS)
Superiority of democracy	3.443	3.292	3.638	3.506	77.897*** (CRS>LDS=RES>RIS)
General trust	3.136	3.240	3.407	3.479	29.685*** (RES=CRS>LDS=RIS)
Political system efficiency	4.113	3.872	4.938	4.844	177.147*** (CRS=RES>LDS>RIS)

Note: *<.05, **<.01, ***<.001.

They do not believe that democracy is superior, they oppose emergency protocols, and they do not think their nation's democratic system works well. When the findings are considered collectively, it can be concluded that East Asians generally favor limited government. The variations based on particular indices are explained below.

East Asians who support a Liberal Democratic State place a high value on personal freedom and personal accountability, which is why they are more likely to see COVID-19-related damage as owing to personal responsibility rather than to random events. On the other hand, those who support a Communitarian Regulative State typically view "bad luck" as accountable for COVID-19 damage. People who support both the Communitarian Regulative State and the Rule by Order Exceptional State generally have a lot in common. They are more inclined than other categories of citizens to support strict restrictions on entry into the country by foreigners and substantial government financial assistance for victims. They have strong nationalism and authoritarian tendencies, and support the government's strict COVID-19 quarantine policy. However, it is interesting to note that the supporters of the Communitarian Regulative State show higher support for "superiority of democracy" than the supporters of the Liberal Democratic State.

However, there are also a lot of commonalities among those who support a Liberal Democratic State or a Rule of Law Intervention State—that is, they all value individual liberty. They embrace little nationalism or authoritarianism and are rather apathetic toward the COVID-19 tight quarantine laws, economic support initiatives, and strict restrictions on entry into the country by foreigners. Additionally, there is a propensity to resist the government's implementation of strict emergency protocols.

However, it is crucial to note that directly comparing index differences based on governance type can be difficult because each index has its own unique scale. As a result, the ten indices underwent standardization and expression as a visual graph, with the outcomes displayed in Figure 8.2.

The standardized indices were compared to determine the impact of the four COVID-19 governance models. One can see that the two models—Liberal Democratic State and Rule of Law Intervention State—share a similar slope in the lower half of Figure 8.2, as do the Communitarian Regulative State and the Rule by Order Exceptional State models in the upper half. The index showing the widest degree of disparity among the four governance types was "strict emergency protocols." Support for the government's extreme emergency measures ranged, as follows, from high to low: Communitarian Regulative State, Rule by Order Exceptional State, Liberal Democratic State, and Rule of Law Intervention State. When seen as a whole, the Communitarian Regulative State and Rule of Law Intervention State models exhibit starkly divergent viewpoints about strict COVID-19 protocols and are situated at opposite extremities of the cross-tabulation of governance types. Despite ranking next-to-lowest of the indices in terms of support for protocols, the Liberal Democratic State exhibits the strongest belief that individuals bear responsibility for the damage suffered from COVID-19.

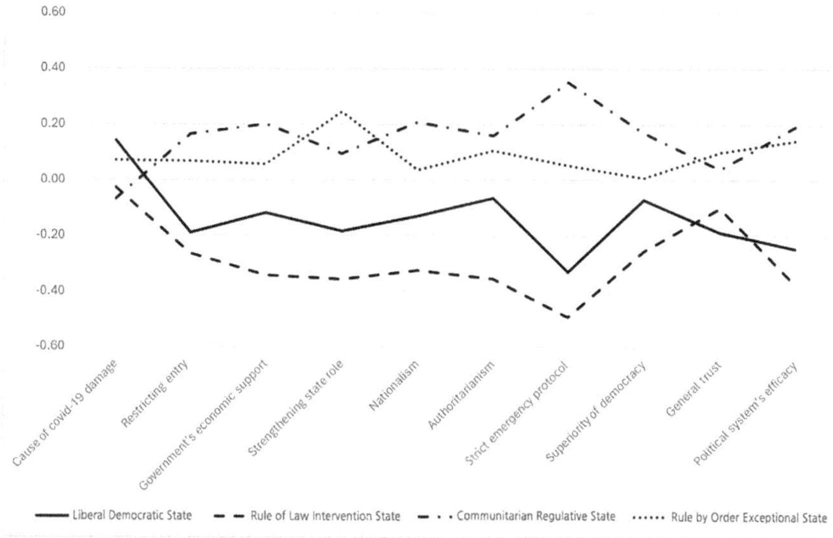

Figure 8.2 Index by governance types. (please stretch figure 8.2 to the right direction in Figure 8.1.

An Evaluative Comparison of Responses to COVID-19 in Japan, South Korea, and China

This research's first section examined East Asia through the eyes of global citizens. It was mentioned that East Asians are highly competitive with one another, highly sensitive, and at times overcritical, hence they are often very stingy when it comes to praising their neighbor countries. I now want to focus on East Asia and use data analysis to examine this problem through two investigations: The first is how the people of the three East Asian countries assess the effectiveness of the COVID-19 quarantine enforced by the governments of Japan, South Korea, and China. The second concerns the assessment of citizens from the three East Asian nations of the degree to which the governments of China, Japan, and Korea have attempted to foster international collaboration on the quarantine issue during the global spread of COVID-19.

The questionnaires we employed are as follows:

(1) "Do you agree that the following state/region/organization has done a good job dealing with the coronavirus outbreak?" After reading the question, respondents were asked to rank their agreement on a scale of 1 to 5 with the assertion that each government has achieved highly positive quarantine results, notably mentioning China, Korea, and Japan.
(2) "Do you agree that the following state contributes to international cooperation to reduce coronavirus cases?" After reading the question, respondents

were asked to use the same methodology to rank the accomplishments of the governments of China, Korea, and Japan on a scale from 1 to 5.

Data analysis shows that the COVID-19 quarantine performance of the governments of China, Japan, and Korea was evaluated by their respective populations as being noticeably better than that of other nations. When comparing the disparities by nation, Japanese citizens thought that all three countries' quarantine efforts were about the same, but that the Japanese government performed better. In contrast, Chinese citizens thought that their government performed far better than any other country. Korean citizens, too, thought their government performed noticeably better than that of other countries. Based on the evaluative rankings, Chinese respondents stated that China, Korea, and Japan fared well in that order, whereas Korean respondents stated that Korea, Japan, and China performed well in that order. Figure 8.3 presents a clearer picture of the difference.

The average of the quarantine assessments, as provided by the citizens of China, Korea, and Japan, respectively, is denoted by the number 0 in Figure 8.3, which serves as the benchmark for comparison. Based on this average, each bar represents the degree to which the quarantine performance differs from the benchmark (0). Japanese citizens perceived the government of their country to have performed fairly well when compared to the three East Asian countries' average performance; however, they rated the Chinese and Korean governments' performance as below average. This indicates that, although the degree of superiority is not so very high, Japanese citizens believed their government handled the COVID-19 quarantine better than any other East Asian country. On the other hand, Chinese citizens rated Japan's quarantine performance as appalling, while rating their own government's

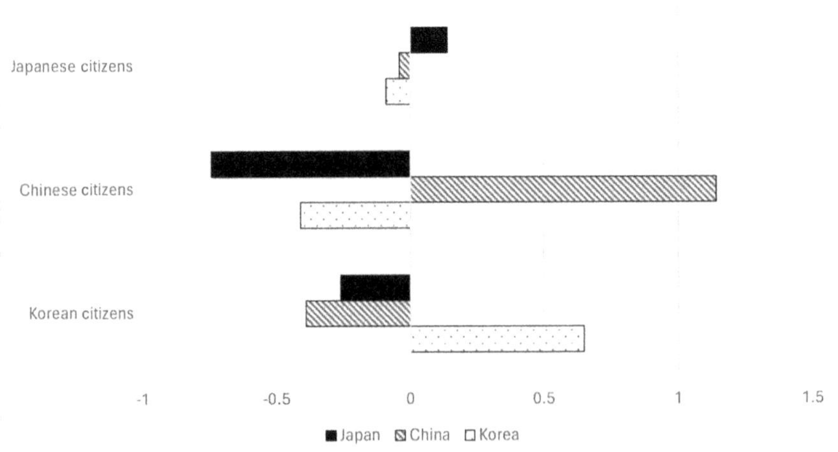

Figure 8.3 Quarantine competence (bar graph).

performance as noticeably better than that of other East Asian countries. In the eyes of Chinese citizens, the Korean government's performance was also below average. In Korea, the nationalist-centered approach functioned similarly. Korean citizens thought that the Korean government performed significantly better when it comes to quarantining Korean citizens than the average of the three East Asian countries; on the other hand, they thought that the Chinese government performed significantly worse than the average, and while they thought that the Japanese government performed better than China, Japan still fell short of the average.

Similar tendencies can be seen in assessments of international collaboration, with the highest value placed on the contribution of one's own nation. In terms of international collaboration to prevent COVID-19, Korean citizens assessed the Korean government as being the most active, Chinese citizens the Chinese government, and Japanese citizens the Japanese government. While Korean, Chinese, and Japanese citizens all exhibit the same nationalist-centered tendency, it was discovered that Chinese citizens exhibited it to a significantly greater extent than Korean citizens.

Based on the data collected, an objective assessment of the three East Asian countries' COVID-19 quarantine performance and their role in fostering international collaboration may be made. A significant difference exists between the opinions of Korean, Chinese, and Japanese citizens and the results of this impartial assessment. Evaluations by Chinese citizens in particular clearly exhibited a tendency toward ethnocentrism. But Chinese nationals clearly were not the only ones following this trend. All three of the East Asian countries exhibited this tendency.

Based on these findings, the research now aims to investigate the variations among the ten indices categorized by form of governance.

A Comparison of the Indices for China, Japan, and Korea

The averages of the ten indices for the citizens of Korea, China, and Japan were compared using one-way ANOVA and Scheffe's post hoc test. Table 8.3 presents the analysis results.

China ranked highest while Japan ranked lowest in the majority of the indices. The "cause of COVID-19 damage" index revealed the opposite outcome, with China demonstrating a notable propensity to attribute the virus to "bad luck" as opposed to personal accountability. In summary, the findings show that the Chinese generally supported tighter immigration laws, financial assistance from the government for victims, and increased government intervention. They embraced forceful measures during emergencies and placed a high emphasis on nationalism and authoritarianism. Attitudes regarding democracy were strongest in China as well, similar to Korea. To visually verify the variations in the index between countries, Figure 8.4 was created using standardized indices.

The graph's most variable indices are "causes of COVID-19 harm" and "political system efficiency." Whereas Japanese and Korean citizens were more likely to ascribe harm from COVID-19 to individual carelessness, Chinese citizens strongly tended to blame "bad luck," likely because collectivism is more common

Table 8.3 Index by three countries (stretch table 8.3 to the right direction as in Table 8.1 and 8.2

	K *(Korea)*	*C* *(China)*	*J* *(Japan)*	*F* *(Scheffe)*
Cause of Covid-19 damage	5.44	3.48	5.35	1378.85*** (K=J>C)
Entry restrictions	3.48	3.75	3.51	23.39*** (C>K=J)
Government support	3.09	3.87	2.76	397.86*** (C>K>J)
Strengthening state role	3.95	4.11	3.52	206.89*** (C>K>J)
Nationalism	5.33	5.45	4.83	126.76*** (C>K>J)
Authoritarianism	5.58	5.73	5.16	58.08*** (C>K>J)
Strict emergency protocols	4.66	5.28	4.25	190.05*** (C>K>J)
Superiority of democracy	3.67	3.69	3.15	156.64*** (J>K=C)
General trust	3.20	3.80	3.07	190.05*** (C>K>J)
Political system efficiency	4.38	5.94	3.40	156.64*** (C=K>J)

Note: *<.05, **<.01, ***<.001.

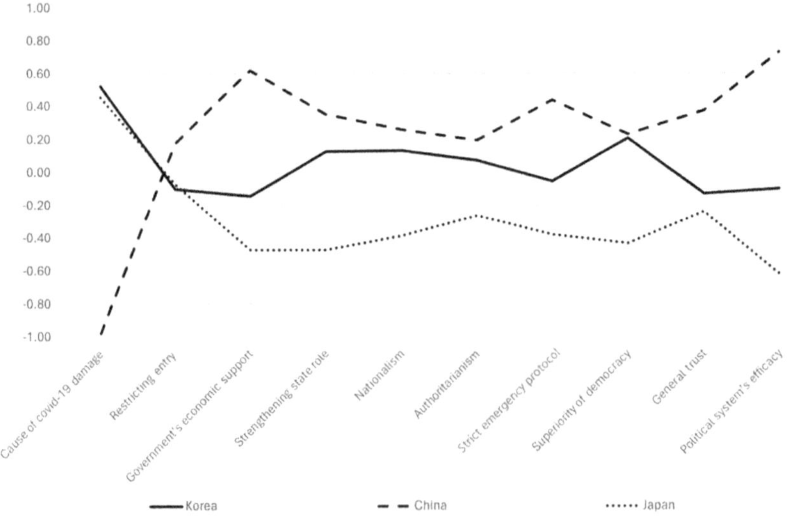

Figure 8.4 Index by three countries. Stretch figure 8.4 in the same way.

than individuality in Chinese society. "Political system efficiency" pertains to the assessment made by the populace regarding how their respective political systems handled the tasks of disease inspection, quarantine, management, and eradication in reaction to the COVID-19 crisis. Figure 8.4 illustrates how the Chinese thought the Chinese government was extremely efficient, the Japanese thought the Japanese government was underdeveloped, and the Koreans thought the Korean government was somewhere in the middle between China and Japan in terms of efficiency in managing the pandemic.

Responses to the "entry restrictions" index showed that the three countries shared remarkably similar views on emergency border control. It was predicted that the indices pertaining to COVID-19 performance would be different in China vis-à-vis Japan and Korea due to disparities in the countries' political and economic systems. However, as this study's results demonstrate, China and Korea were most similar, while Japan exhibited significant divergence with the exception of just a few indices.

Effect of Each Index on Assessing Political System Efficiency

Next, the research will use "political system efficiency" as the dependent variable, and search for independent factors that influence it, since it has been demonstrated to have a substantial impact on citizens' consciousness and assessments in the three East Asian countries. OLS regression analysis was carried out for this purpose. Table 8.4 presents the analysis results.

Table 8.4 OLS regression toward political system efficiency Stretch in the same way

	Total	*Korean*	*Chinese*	*Japanese*
Age	−0.004*	0.001	−0.005	−0.004
Gender (0=Female)				
Male	−0.026	−0.092	0.050	−0.088
Subjective class	0.098***	0.308***	−0.032	−0.013
Cause of Covid-19 damage	0.054*	−0.081	0.148***	−0.013
Entry restrictions	−0.142***	−0.223***	−0.011	−0.045
Government support	0.582***	0.500***	0.369***	0.692***
Strengthening state role	0.192***	0.239**	0.377***	−0.121*
Nationalism	0.205***	0.125	0.085*	0.150*
Authoritarianism	−0.065***	−0.252***	0.319***	−0.083*
Strict emergency protocols	0.282***	0.380***	0.136**	0.177***
Superiority of democracy	0.011	0.064	−0.018	0.148*
General trust	0.136***	0.151***	0.113***	0.137***
Country (0=South Korean)				
Chinese	0.928***			
Japanese	−0.431***			
Constant	−0.596*	0.457	−0.634	0.482
Adjusted R^2	0.530	0.385	0.424	0.333
N	3,000	1,000	1,000	1,000

Note: *<.05, **<.01, ***<.001.

Examining the three East Asian countries collectively, it appears that the older the population, the more likely it is that they will perceive the political system in their country as being less effective. When it comes to subjective class consciousness, the more highly someone values their social standing, the higher they will assess the efficiency of their country's political system. Examining the effects of each index, it was discovered that all but the "democracy" index had a statistically significant impact on assessments of "political system efficiency." There may be some correlation between the assessment of a country's political system and its level of democracy. Democratic countries like Japan and Korea are perceived as having comparably positive images, but China is opposite. It was established through international comparison that Japan's political system was regarded as more efficient the more favorable its democratic system was viewed. "Authoritarianism" and "entry restrictions" are two indices that showed a negative correlation with "political system efficiency." Those who believed that active entry restrictions are required also generally believed that the political system in their country is inefficient. Likewise, the more their appreciation for authoritarianism, the more inefficient they believed their country's political system to be. In fact, based on values by country, China's political system was rated as being more effective the more authoritarian the rating country was; conversely, a negative correlation was found between China and Korea. As was previously established, when breaking down the disparities by nation, China gave its country the highest ratings overall, followed by Korea and Japan.

When examining the results by country, Chinese citizens perceived a political system to be more efficient the more financial support the government provides for COVID-19 victims. According to this line of reasoning, a powerful state serves to maintain the efficiency of the political system. The political system is seen as more efficient the higher its authoritarianism score. Furthermore, the greater the belief among individuals that the harm caused by COVID-19 is the victim's own responsibility, the more efficient they viewed their nation's political system.

In the instance of Korea, citizens viewed political sanctions to be more effective the greater their subjective class attribution. The perception of the political system's efficiency in enacting robust emergency protocols was positively correlated with the level of government support for victims. The political system was thought to be more inefficient the higher the authoritarianism rating. Generally speaking, the political system was viewed as more efficient the higher the level of confidence in the system. The perception of the political system's inefficiency increased with the implementation of stricter limits on entry restrictions by foreigners.

The regression analysis findings in the case of Japan resembled those of Korea. What is interesting, though, is that it was discovered that "political system efficiency" was negatively impacted by "strong government role." The political system was viewed as less effective the more value was placed on authoritarianism. From the overall results, it may be concluded that, out of the three East Asian countries, the political system in Japan is the most removed from authoritarianism. This is significant. The political system was viewed as more efficient the stronger the citizens believed in democracy. It appears that the Japanese consider their government to be a far cry from authoritarianism and to be a model of well-executed democracy.

Concluding Remarks

The main findings of this comparative study of Japan, South Korea, and China concerning the evaluation of the COVID-19 quarantine performance can be summed up as follows.

(1) The citizens of Japan, Korea, and China are all highly ethnocentric when evaluating the government performance of the three countries reciprocally. This tendency is particularly strong in China followed by Korea and Japan.
(2) Confronting the challenge of COVID-19 pandemic, the most preferred type of governance by East Asian citizens is a Communitarian Regulative State which combines community orientation and individual initiative. This type is clearly distinguished from both Liberal Democratic State and Rule by Order Exceptional State. However, the preference for the Rule by Order Exceptional State is quite high in China compared with Korea and Japan.
(3) Concerning the ten indices created in this chapter, data analysis has demonstrated significant relationships between the four types of governance and these indices. In particular, Liberal Democratic State and Rule of Law Intervention State share a similar pattern, as do the Communitarian Regulative State and the Rule by Order Exceptional State. The contrasting slope of the former in the lower half of the figure while the slope of the latter in the upper half shows this finding clearly.
(4) The national comparison of the indices has shown that Chinese generally support tighter immigration laws, financial assistance from the government for victims, and increased government intervention. They embrace forceful measures during emergencies and placed a high emphasis on nationalism and authoritarianism.
(5) Finally, the regression analysis has shown that the political system was viewed as less effective the more value was placed on authoritarianism. From the overall results, it may be concluded that, out of the three East Asian countries, the political system in Japan is the most removed from authoritarianism. The political system is viewed as more efficient the stronger the citizens believed in democracy.

Notes

1 The basic information of this survey and the main findings of the national characteristics of each country is available in the Website of Joongmin Foundation: www.joongmin.org.
2 Joongmin Foundation, in fact, conducted the first global survey in May 2020 over 30 global cities and offered media briefings in June at Korea Press Center in Seoul, addressing to such salient issues as "the rise of a Korean Model and its Hidden danger," "the collapse

of the United States Hegemony from a global perspective," "Japan at the crossroad with frustrated citizens," and "the divided global images of China."

3 This methodology can eliminate the collective biases that we frequently face when attempting international comparison. These biases are related to cultural dispositive of nations and people. For instance, some people are very lenient in their evaluation, while others are very harsh. We can eliminate such biases by taking a country's specific world average as a standard for its specific international comparison.

References

Agamben, Girogio. 2005. *State of Exception*. Chicago: University of Chicago Press.

Boeing, Philipp, and Yihan Wang. 2021. Decoding China's CPVOD-19 "virus exceptionalism": Community-based digital contact tracing in Wuhan. *R & D Management* 51(4): 339–351.

Degerman, Dan. 2020. The political is medical now: COVID-19, medicalization and political theory. *Theory and Event* 23(4): 61–75.

Domingues, Jose Marricio. 2022. From global risk to global threat: State capabilities and modernity in times of coronavirus. *Current Sociology* 70(1): 6–23.

Han, Qide. 2020. Introduction: The COVID-19 pandemic calls for the strengthening of scientific culture. *Cultures of Science* 3(4): 223–226.

Han, Sang-jin. 2020a. *Confucianism and Reflexive Modernity: Bringing Community Back to Human Rights in the Age of Global Risk Society*. Leiden: Brill.

Han, Sang-jin. 2020b. The future of Korea in post-COVID19 era. In Lee Yonghan et al. (eds.,), *Post-COVID19 Korea*, Seoul: Hanwool, pp. 66–82 (in Korean).

Han, Sang-jin. 2020c. COVID19 Quarantine and the metamorphosis of national image. In Lee Yonghan et al. (eds.), *Post-COVID19 Korea*, Seoul: Hanwool, pp. 98–112 (in Korean).

Han, Sang-jin. 2023. COVID-19 and hegemonic modernity: Post-Western sociological imagination. In Laurence Roulleau-Berger, Li Peilin, Kim Seung Kuk, and Yazawa Shujiro (eds.), *Handbook of Post-Western Sociology: From East Asia to Europe*, Leiden: Brill, pp. 306–325.

He, Alex Jingwei, Yoda Shi, and Hongdou Liu. 2020. Crisis governance, Chinese Style: Distinctive features of China's response to the COVID-19 pandemic. *Policy Design and Practice* 3(3): 242–258.

Hillenbrand, Margaret. 2010. Communitarianism, or, how to build East Asian theory. *Postcolonial Studies* 13(4): 317–334.

Hosoda, Miwako. 2023. Health disparity and global human health from sociological perspective. A paper presented at the conference on modernization and post-modernization: Comparisons and prospects of social development in East Asia held in Jilin University, Changchun. August 11–13.

Jing, Yijia. 2021. Seeking opportunities from crisis? China's governance responses to the COVID-19 pandemic. *International Review of Administrative Sciences* 87(3): 631–650.

Prasad, Amit. 2022. Anti-science misinformation and conspiracies: COVID-19, post-truth, and science & technology studies. *Science, Technology & Society* 27(1): 88–112.

Rolland, Nadege. 2020. China's pandemic power play. *Journal of Democracy* 31(3): 25–38.

Schnitt, Carl. 1934. *Politische Theologie: Vier Kapital zur Lehre von der Souveränität*. Berlin: Dunker & Humblot.

Shim, Young-he e. 2023. Two contradictory trends in Korea in the COVID-19 era: Condensed radicalization of individualization and community orientation. A paper presented at the conference on modernization and post-modernization: Comparisons and prospects of social development in East Asia held in Jilin University, Changchun. August 11–13.

Sprong, Stefanie, Jolanda Jetten, Zhechen Wang, Kim Peters, et al. 2019. "Our country needs a strong leader right now": Economic inequality enhances the wish for a strong leader. *Psychological Science* 30(11): 1625–1637.

Wang, Peter. 2022. *What Do the Chinese Think about Their Government's Response to COVID-19?* Chicago Council on Global Affairs. January 13.

9 Access to Information and Approval of Domestic and Neighboring Countries' Pandemic Responses

Yida Zhai

Introduction

Due to different political and cultural contexts, each country responded to the COVID-19 pandemic in its own way. Initially, some countries sought to disguise the outbreak of the disease and suppressed their citizens' alarm over this public health crisis, while other countries took speedy measures to respond to the spread of infection. Thanks to advanced medical technologies, humans may reduce the harmful outcomes of viruses to some extent but are unable to eliminate all viruses. In fact, viruses evolve and coexist with human society. After COVID-19 had overwhelmed global health systems, some countries treated the pandemic as a public health disaster, one that was not unprecedented in human history. They implemented a social distancing policy, promoted effective vaccination, and imposed restrictions on social gatherings and activities to control the spread of the virus. In contrast, some countries politicized the COVID-19 pandemic for an instrumental purpose. The governments of those countries sought to demonstrate their superior performance in infection prevention and control and the superiority of their political systems. Therefore, they pursued the objective of achieving zero infection, prioritizing it over people's welfare to advance the political leaders' interests. As a result, ordinary people endured significant hardships. Obviously, the government has to persuade people to tolerate unpleasant and painful reality and to believe their country performs well in addressing the COVID-19 pandemic.

Citizens' approval of the government's anti-pandemic response matters for government turnover and the changing relationship between citizens and the state. People's evaluations are not merely based on the actual performance of the government; they also involve other factors. Chapter 4 discussed the two types of political culture. Using the cultural approach, we can explain variations in citizens' approval of the government's response to the pandemic. In liberal cultures, people are more critical of the government's performance, whereas in paternalist cultures, people tend to evaluate their government more favorably (Pye, 1968). In addition, the information environment affects people's evaluations of each country's response to the pandemic. In modern society, information plays a relevant role in shaping public opinion; hence, this chapter explains the role of information in shaping varying popular evaluations of the government's response to the pandemic. It

DOI: 10.4324/9781003495239-12

employs the theoretical framework of an information environment, which includes information from the media and interpersonal networks.

Beyond national borders, citizens also perceive and evaluate other countries' responses to the COVID-19 pandemic. This chapter explores the relationship between citizens' access to information in China, Japan, and South Korea and their approval of the pandemic response of domestic and neighboring countries. It is unclear how the information environment in each country affects people's evaluations of other countries' anti-pandemic performance. Was the information environment in China, Japan, and South Korea critical of or favorable to their neighboring countries? The present study compares Chinese, Japanese, and South Korean citizens' perceptions of their own countries' responses to the pandemic and analyzes how they view their neighboring countries' performance in tackling the pandemic. The results indicate the similarities and differences between these three countries.

Information Environment: The Media and Interpersonal Networks

How citizens evaluate their domestic and neighboring countries' anti-pandemic response may be influenced by the information they have access to. The existing literature divides the information environment into two broad types: information from the media and information from interpersonal networks (First et al., 2021; Han and Zhai, 2022; Scheufele et al., 2004; Richey and Ikeda, 2006). For health communication, these two channels remain the predominant information sources in a public health crisis, and people often acquire information from multiple sources (Jang and Baek, 2019; Spence et al., 2007). Specifically, the transmission of information through the media is unconstrained by distance and can be accessed as long as users have access to media. Nevertheless, information circulating in interpersonal networks is restricted to people's various relationships with others, and the characteristics of these personal relationships determine the availability of this type of information. Regardless of the source of the media or interpersonal networks, information can help people better address crises, but too much exposure to information was observed to be associated with fear and anxiety (Fukasawa et al., 2021; Silver et al., 2013; Thompson et al., 2017).

The media is the primary information source for people in modern societies. Studies stress the media's role in contributing to and intensifying polarization in people's worldviews (Morris, 2007). In particular, in past decades, the populist media has fabricated news and manipulated public grievance in the midst of the backlash against multiculturalism (Castle, 2011). Mass media, such as newspapers, television, and radio, had dominated the information environment in the 20th century. Despite the development of digital technologies, empirical studies show that the mass media continues to be a powerful medium and can influence people's attitudes (Anderson 2006; Guo and Wang, 2021; Han and Zhai, 2022; Yang et al., 2014). Mass media frames the presentation of an issue, constructs the meanings, and molds public sentiment (Bednarek and Caple, 2017; Fiss and Hirsch, 2005). Although people can select their exposure to different sources of information, they are primarily receivers of information when using mass media. The information transmission is unidirectional from media agencies to users.

Differing from mass media, the internet and social media involve multiple sources of content such as text, images, and video. They provide global and instant information as well as interactive communication. Social media makes access to information easier and provides diverse perspectives on the same issue (Chung and Fu, 2022; Xiang and Hmielowski, 2017). Transmission of information becomes speedy and instantaneous; an event can be simultaneously displayed online as if it happened in front of viewers. Social media users are not passive receivers of information but become active senders of information (Zhai, 2021). Everyone is able to express their voices on the internet or through social media and exchange ideas online. This is a two-way communication process. Some studies have found that disinformation or false information is easier to circulate on the internet and social media (Gao et al., 2020).

Interpersonal networks provide people with alternative information channels that are different from media channels. Transmission of information occurs through the communication process, including casual talks or formal discussions (Ikeda and Richey, 2005; Monge and Contractor, 2003; Weimann, 1983). Communication in interpersonal networks is a normal way to exchange and share information in people's everyday lives. People can access information through communication with kins, friends, neighbors, coworkers, or other members of NGOs (Boase and Ikeda, 2012; Ikeda and Boase, 2011; Scheufele et al., 2004). Information from this type of channel is often informal and mixes with personal experience or grapevines, but it provides additional information beyond official channels (Jang and Baek, 2019). During the pandemic, interpersonal networks are important information sources.

The information environment in China is different from that in Japan and South Korea. For the latter two countries, media markets mainly comprise private media agencies, and both liberal and conservative media information exists (Chrisman, 2008; Chung et al., 2021). A single media agency can rarely dominate public opinion. Instead, many media organizations compete to report an issue from different perspectives and stances; accordingly, Japan and South Korea showed a greater diversity of opinions in the media. In contrast, China's authoritarian state imposes censorship on the media and determines what information people can access. The types of information sources individuals use influence their evaluations of each country's response to the pandemic at home and abroad. China's mass media is strictly controlled by government authorities, and the information in mass media tends to serve government interests (Guo and Wang, 2021; Yang, 2013; Zhu, 2014). In terms of China's pandemic propaganda, mass media often praises China's "successful response to COVID-19," while stressing the flaws or incompetence of other countries by contending that Western-style democracy performed poorly in controlling infection (Zhai, 2023b, 2024; Zhai et al., 2022).

Although Chinese authorities can monopolize domestic mass media through carrot-and-stick policies, it is difficult to gain complete control of the internet. Censorship agencies at different levels of government have diversified their aims and incentives, which leads to a fragmented system of internet regulation (Tai, 2014). Therefore, internet censorship is selective and leaves some room for the expression of different opinions (Chi, 2012; Yang, 2013). In contrast to the mass media's flattery of the country's anti-pandemic performance, Chinese citizens can access information that questions or criticizes the zero-COVID policy on the internet. Indeed, this policy has led to heated online debates, indicating that different opinions coexist online. Therefore, the internet is considered an important outlet for liberals to express their opinions in China.

Variations in Access to Information in the Three Countries

This section empirically examines the characteristics of access to information on the COVID-19 pandemic in China, Japan, and South Korea. The content of the information in the three countries focused on different themes, such as infection prevention, economic downturn, social welfare, and governance during the pandemic (Lee et al., 2020; Parvin et al., 2022; Zhao et al., 2021). Our survey asked respondents in the three countries how frequently they obtained information on COVID-19 from a list of sources. Information sources were categorized into two broad types: the media (newspapers, television, the internet, and social media) and interpersonal networks (family members, friends, and colleagues). Frequency of access to the above information sources was measured on a five-point scale, from 1 "not at all" to 5 "every day." Figure 9.1 presents the results of access to information in the three countries.

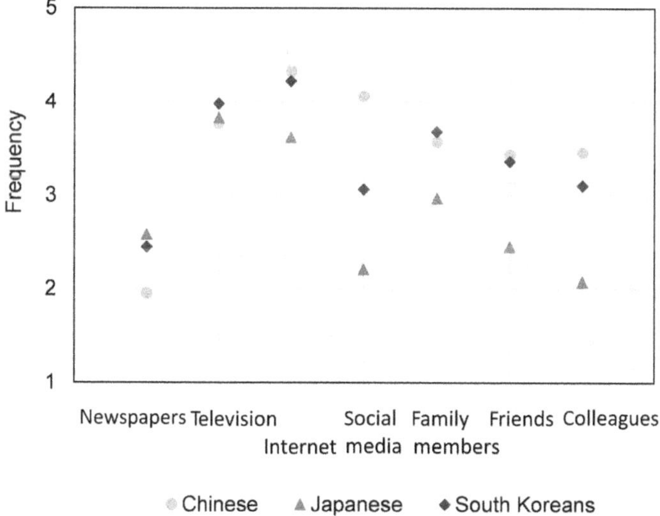

Figure 9.1 Comparison of access to information regarding the pandemic across the three countries.

In China, people's most frequently accessed information sources were television, the internet, social media, and family. The influence of newspapers in China has indeed decreased, and newspapers were the least frequently used source for acquiring information on COVID-19. However, even with the decline in traditional media, television remains a major source of information for Chinese people, as seen in Figure 9.1. The frequency with which information was acquired from family members, friends, and colleagues was almost on a similar level, revealing the characteristics of Chinese people's interpersonal relationships. Friends and colleagues were as important as family members in their exchange of and access to information on COVID-19.

In Japan, the primary sources of information on COVID-19 were television, the internet, and family members. Japanese people also used newspapers as a source of information, but they tended not to rely on colleagues as a source of information on COVID-19. The Japanese working environment might not encourage interpersonal communication among staff about work-irrelevant issues. Among interpersonal networks, family was the most frequent information channel for Japanese people, followed by networks of friends. The degree of closeness of the relationships in personal networks determined the frequency of access to a certain source of information.

In South Korea, the main means of access to information on COVID-10 were television, the internet, and family. South Korea was similar in this respect to Japan. Newspapers were not the primary information source either. Frequency of access to information from interpersonal networks was consistent with the degree of closeness of the relationship. Family was the most frequently used source of information on COVID-19; networks of friends came second. Users enjoyed less frequent access to information from colleagues than from family and friends. A similar pattern was observed in Japan, but the degree of difference in the frequency of South Korean citizens' access to information between these interpersonal relationships was smaller than that in Japan.

The findings indicate the degree to which access to information on the COVID-19 pandemic varies across the three countries, reflecting the different media environments and social relationships in these three countries.

Ingroup Favoritism and Evaluations of Domestic and Foreign Responses to the Pandemic

Social identity theory states that people construct their self-concepts partially based on their membership in a social group (Tajfel, 1982; Tajfel and Turner, 1986). They divide the world into ingroups and outgroups and conform their social identity to the ingroup. People tend to perceive and emphasize similarities of ingroup members but exaggerate the differences between ingroups and outgroups. Social categorization between "us" and "them" shapes different attitudinal and behavioral responses to members of ingroups and outgroups. Studies demonstrate that the construction of social identity creates a tendency toward ingroup favoritism (Tajfel, 1974; Tajfel and Turner, 1986). People are prone to evaluate their ingroups more favorably or award more resources to their ingroup members (Efferson et al., 2008; Fisher, 1990; Romano et al., 2017). Social psychologists have found that this ingroup bias even exists in groups temporarily and randomly divided according to certain arbitrary criteria, in situations in which group members actually share minimal common characteristics. Social identity theory has been widely used to explain prejudice, discrimination, and intergroup conflict.

China, Japan, and South Korea have a long history of mutual interaction, marked not only by friendly cultural exchange but also by conflicts and wars. Even today, quarrels occur and escalate to conflicts over the history of World War II, territorial disputes, Japanese politicians' visits to the Yasukuni Shrine, comfort women, hanbok, and kimchee. Even a trivial issue can arouse heated debate. Under the influence of these historical and current disagreements, ordinary people in the three countries also view each other unfavorably (The Genron NPO, 2021). Citizens' evaluation of their domestic and neighboring countries' responses to the pandemic may be affected by the tendency to favor their national ingroups.

The present study examined citizens' approval of domestic and neighboring countries' responses to the pandemic. Our survey asked respondents whether anti-pandemic measures in China, Japan, and South Korea were successful or unsuccessful. Their responses were coded on a 5-point scale, and the higher scores indicated more favorable evaluations. Figure 9.2 shows the results. Ingroup favoritism had the greatest salience among Chinese citizens. They gave China a score of 4.611 on a 5-point scale but gave fairly low evaluations to Japan and South Korea. In their eyes, China performed much better than the other two countries. South Korean citizens also showed a similar tendency. They evaluated South Korea more favorably than China and Japan, and of the nationals of all three countries, they gave the neighboring countries the lowest scores. Ingroup favoritism was the

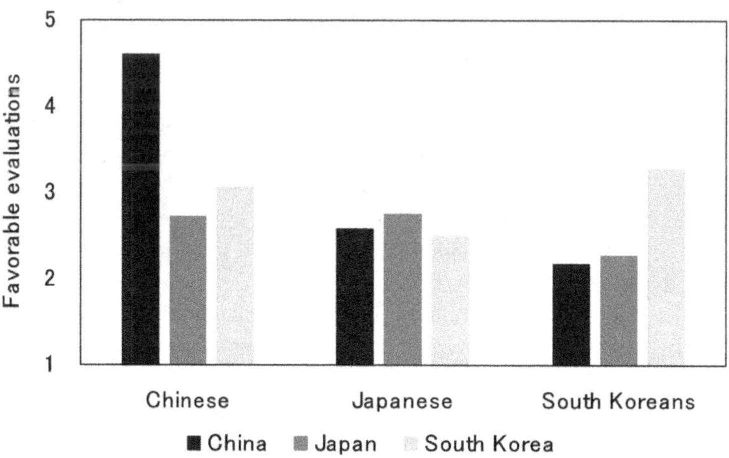

Figure 9.2 Evaluations of domestic and foreign responses to the pandemic.

weakest in Japan. Japanese citizens scored Japan only slightly higher than China and South Korea. On a 5-point scale, the median was 3 points, but none of the countries' average scores were higher than that, indicating that Japanese people evaluated all three countries negatively.

These results show that citizens of all three East Asian countries tend to favor their ingroup; this social psychological tendency is strongest in China and much weaker in Japan. Differences in political cultures and systems may account for this difference. Japan's democratic system allows people to express criticism of the authorities, and ordinary people have been used to criticizing the government. However, China's authoritarian political system does not tolerate criticism from its citizens, and approval of the government is political correctness. In addition, nationalism is prevalent in China, and Chinese nationalists consider China to be superior to other nations. Clearly, this mentality influences their evaluations of China's response to the pandemic and that of other countries. South Koreans' tendency toward ingroup favoritism is in between that of the Chinese and that of the Japanese. They tend to evaluate their own country more favorably than others, but not to the same extreme extent as in China.

Access to Information and Chinese Citizens' Approval of the Domestic and Foreign Responses to the Pandemic

This section examines the relationships between access to different sources of information and Chinese citizens' evaluations of national responses to the pandemic in China, Japan, and Korea. Figure 9.2 reveals that Chinese citizens had extraordinarily high evaluations of China but low evaluations of the two neighboring countries. It is unclear whether an intergenerational difference existed in this pattern of evaluations or whether it was universal among Chinese of all age groups. The relationship between generations and evaluations of the countries' response to the pandemic was first examined. The original scale for evaluating the countries' anti-pandemic responses consisted of five points. For ease of comparison, the present study integrated the categories of "very successful" and "somewhat successful" into the category of "successful," and the categories of "very unsuccessful" and "somewhat unsuccessful" into the category of "unsuccessful." Therefore, the following analysis used a three-category variable to evaluate the three countries' anti-pandemic responses. Table 9.1 presents the results of the contingency table analysis using two categorical variables: generations (18–30 years old, 31–50 years old, and 51 and above) and evaluations of countries' anti-pandemic response (unsuccessful, neutral, and successful).

The results show that how Chinese citizens evaluated China's response to the pandemic was not independent from the generations to which they belonged, $\chi^2 = 20.557$, $p < 0.001$. Younger Chinese evaluated their own country more favorably. Among respondents 18 to 30 years of age, 97.19% had a favorable evaluation of China. This age group of Chinese strongly supported the country's anti-pandemic response. Conversely, the older generations had greater reservations about China's performance than their younger counterparts. Uncritical attitudes toward the state

Table 9.1 Variations in Chinese citizens' evaluations of domestic and foreign responses to the pandemic across different generations

		Evaluations of the responses to the pandemic									*Total*
		China			*Japan*			*South Korea*			
		Unsuccessful	*Neutral*	*Successful*	*Unsuccessful*	*Neutral*	*Successful*	*Unsuccessful*	*Neutral*	*Successful*	
Generations	18–30	4 (1.02%)	7 (1.79%)	380 (97.18%)	137 (35.04%)	189 (48.34%)	65 (16.62%)	76 (19.44%)	209 (53.45%)	106 (27.11%)	391 (39.10%)
	31–50	9 (2.45%)	11 (2.99%)	348 (94.57%)	163 (44.29%)	136 (36.96%)	69 (18.75%)	74 (20.11%)	190 (51.63%)	104 (28.26%)	368 (36.80%)
	51–	17 (7.05%)	5 (2.07%)	219 (90.87%)	92 (38.17%)	98 (40.66%)	51 (21.16%)	52 (21.58%)	120 (49.79%)	69 (28.63%)	241 (24.10%)
	Total	30 (3.00%)	23 (2.30%)	947 (94.70%)	392 (39.20%)	423 (42.30%)	185 (18.50%)	202 (20.20%)	519 (51.90%)	279 (27.90%)	1000 (100%)

among young Chinese went against the change of values predicted by modernization theory, which is a topic worthy of further research.

How Chinese citizens evaluated Japan's response to the pandemic was also contingent on what generation they belonged to, $\chi^2 = 11.913$, $p = 0.018$. Respondents between 31 and 50 years old evaluated Japan's anti-COVID-19 response more negatively. Almost half of the respondents (48.34%) under age 31 evaluated Japan's response to the pandemic neutrally: They did not form an explicitly favorable or unfavorable evaluation of Japan's response.

How Chinese citizens evaluated South Korea's response to the pandemic was independent of the generation to which they belonged, $\chi^2 = 0.884$, $p = 0.927$. Table 9.1 shows that around one-third of respondents evaluated South Korea's pandemic response positively; 50% of respondents took a neutral stance; and 20% of respondents were negative. This pattern of evaluations did not change across different generations and appeared universal among all age groups.

The aforementioned results indicate that favoritism to the national ingroup was stronger among younger Chinese generations. They were more reluctant to criticize China's pandemic response than the older generations. Although Chinese people evaluated Japan's and South Korea's performance in tackling the COVID-19 pandemic unfavorably (see Figure 9.2), evaluations of Japan differed across generations, but the intergenerational variation was not observed in their evaluations of South Korea. Chinese public opinion toward Japan was more diverse than toward South Korea.

Multivariate regression analysis was performed to examine the relationship between Chinese citizens' access to information and their evaluations of domestic and neighboring countries' responses to the pandemic. The demographic attributes such as age, gender, education levels, and income were controlled for in the analysis. Figure 9.3 presents the results of major variables of information sources.

In terms of evaluations of China's response to the pandemic, watching television and internet use were positively associated with the approval of China ($b = 0.115$, $p = 0.001$; $b = 0.334$, $p < 0.001$). In terms of evaluations of Japan's response, social media use was positively associated with Chinese citizens' positive evaluations of Japan's anti-pandemic response ($b = 0.084$, $p = 0.033$). However, neither media information nor information in interpersonal networks was associated with the approval of South Korea's response to the pandemic.

The aforementioned results have two implications. First, information sources provided explanations for Chinese citizens' evaluation of their own country but were not primary factors that influenced the evaluations of Japan's and South Korea's response to the pandemic. Television and the internet might disseminate positive information on China; accordingly, people who accessed information more frequently from these two sources tended to strongly approve of China's anti-pandemic performance. Conversely, R-squared values in the models of evaluations of Japan and South Korea were fairly low, showing that the outcome variables were scarcely explained by access to information. One possible explanation is that Chinese people's negative evaluations of Japan's and South Korea's responses to the pandemic were not based on information about how these two countries tackled

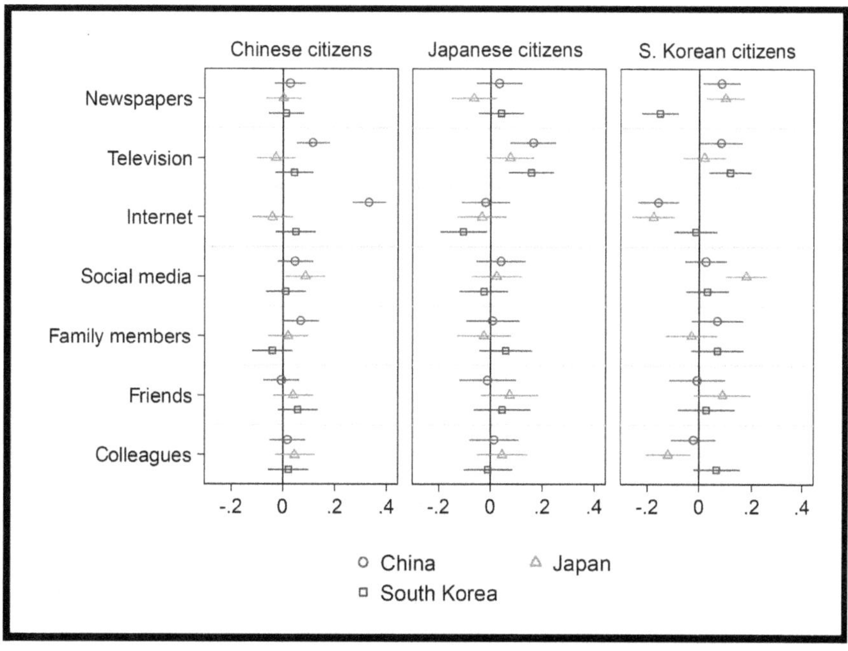

Figure 9.3 Predicting citizens' evaluations of the three countries' pandemic responses.

the pandemic; instead, prejudices toward Japan and South Korea determined their disapproval of the two countries' anti-pandemic responses.

The second implication we can draw from the results is that in China, media information had a greater role in evaluations of China's response to the pandemic than information from interpersonal networks. Although Chinese people also learned about the pandemic from interpersonal networks such as friends and colleagues (see Figure 9.1), this type of information did not significantly affect their evaluations of domestic and foreign countries' anti-pandemic performance. In China, interpersonal communication during the pandemic might focus more on local issues, such as infection, quarantine policy, and shortages of living necessities, rather than national and foreign situations. The latter were covered in the media, such as television, the internet, and social media. The results identified the difference between information in media and information in interpersonal networks in China during the COVID-19 pandemic.

Access to Information and Japanese Citizens' Approval of the Domestic and Foreign Responses to the Pandemic

Using the same method, this section examines the relationships between access to different information sources and Japanese citizens' evaluations of national responses to the pandemic in China, Japan, and Korea. The previous analysis has shown that Japanese citizens were critical of all three countries (including their own country) and evaluated them unfavorably (see Figure 9.2). This section first examines whether this pattern of evaluations varied by different generations. Table 9.2 presents the results of the contingency table analysis. Japanese citizens' evaluation of their own country's response to the pandemic varied by generation, $\chi^2 = 12.270, p = 0.015$. The older generations perceived Japan's response to the pandemic more negatively. One-fifth of younger Japanese favorably evaluated Japan's anti-pandemic response. Younger Japanese show a lower percentage of unfavorable evaluations and a high percentage of neutral stances. A high percentage of neutral responses (48.51%) was recorded among those respondents between 18 and 30 years old; they did not form a clear judgment of Japan's response as being successful or unsuccessful. The results indicate that Japanese young people's evaluations of their own country's performance were in the process of development.

Japanese citizens' evaluations of China's anti-pandemic response also varied across generations, $\chi^2 = 12.939$, $p = 0.012$. The older generations tended to perceive China's performance more positively than their younger counterparts. Those respondents between 31 and 50 years old had the highest percentage of unfavorable evaluations of China's anti-pandemic response. Nearly half of the respondents under age 31 (47.52%) took a neutral stance when evaluating China's response.

Japanese citizens' evaluations of South Korea's anti-pandemic response were independent of the generation to which they belonged, $\chi^2 = 6.293$, $p = 0.178$. Table 9.2 shows that around one-tenth of respondents viewed South Korea's response to the pandemic as successful, 40% of respondents viewed it as unsuccessful, and half of respondents chose a neutral stance. This pattern of evaluations of South Korea's anti-pandemic response did not change significantly across different generations of the Japanese population.

The aforementioned results indicate that although Japanese people disapproved of both China's and South Korea's anti-pandemic responses, there were intergenerational differences in their evaluations of China, but the same tendency was not observed in their evaluations of South Korea. Older generations of Japanese viewed China's zero-COVID policy more favorably than younger ones. Another interesting finding was the neutral stance of Japanese young people, between 18 and 30 years old, in their evaluations of domestic and neighboring countries' anti-pandemic responses. Compared to other generations, they were reluctant to express clear evaluations of these countries' performance during the pandemic.

Multivariate regression analysis was performed to examine the relationship between Japanese people's access to information and their evaluations of domestic and neighboring countries' responses to the pandemic. Similar to the previous analysis of the Chinese case, the analysis controlled for demographic attributes. Figure 9.3 only presents the major results regarding information sources.

In evaluating Japan's response, neither the information from the media nor information from interpersonal networks was significantly associated with the approval of Japan's anti-pandemic response. Access to information from television was positively associated with favorable evaluations of China's response ($b = 0.164$,

Table 9.2 Variations of Japanese citizens' evaluations of domestic and foreign responses to the pandemic across different generations

		Evaluations of the responses to the pandemic									*Total*
		China			*Japan*			*South Korea*			
		Unsuccessful	*Neutral*	*Successful*	*Unsuccessful*	*Neutral*	*Successful*	*Unsuccessful*	*Neutral*	*Successful*	
Generations	18–30	42 (41.58%)	48 (47.52%)	11 (10.89%)	31 (30.69%)	49 (48.51%)	21 (20.79%)	35 (34.65%)	54 (53.47%)	12 (11.88%)	101 (12.52%)
	31–50	123 (46.77%)	108 (41.06%)	32 (12.17%)	103 (39.16%)	105 (39.92%)	55 (20.91%)	115 (43.73%)	131 (49.81%)	17 (6.46%)	263 (32.59%)
	51–	175 (39.50%)	176 (39.73%)	92 (20.77%)	171 (38.60%)	146 (32.96%)	126 (28.44%)	196 (44.24%)	203 (45.82%)	44 (9.93%)	443 (54.89%)
	Total	340 (42.13%)	332 (41.14%)	135 (16.73%)	305 (37.79%)	300 (37.17%)	202 (25.03%)	346 (42.87%)	388 (48.08%)	73 (9.05%)	807 (100%)

$p < 0.001$). Access to information from television was positively associated with favorable evaluations of South Korea's response ($b = 0.156, p = 0.001$), with which internet use was negatively associated ($b = -0.105, p = 0.028$).

The aforementioned results reveal characteristics of the information environment in Japan. First, Japanese people evaluated their own country's performance in tackling the pandemic independently of information they acquired from various sources regardless of the media or interpersonal networks. Figure 9.2 shows that Japanese people disapproved of their country's response to the pandemic. Analysis in this section found that this negative evaluation was not primarily attributable to the information environment. Japanese people might judge their country's response based on their own experiences. They evaluated the effectiveness and costs of the country's anti-pandemic measures; ultimately, they disapproved of Japan's response. Second, contrary to the stereotype that Japanese television is prejudiced against China and South Korea, access to information from television had a positive effect on favorable evaluations of the two neighboring countries' responses to the pandemic. Certainly, this does not mean that Japanese TV stations intended to circulate positive information on China and South Korea. Nevertheless, these two countries' anti-pandemic policies as portrayed in Japanese TV programs earned some approval from Japanese citizens. The adverse effects of these policies might have received more attention in China and South Korea than in Japan.

Access to Information and South Korean Citizens' Approval of the Domestic and Foreign Responses to the Pandemic

Access to information may also influence South Korean citizens' evaluations of national responses to the pandemic in China, Japan, and South Korea. The previous analysis has shown that the presence of favoritism to the national ingroup in terms of evaluations of the country's anti-pandemic response among South Korean citizens (see Figure 9.2). They evaluated South Korea's pandemic response more favorably than those of the two neighboring countries. This section began by examining whether this pattern of evaluation was prevalent in different age groups. Table 9.3 presents the results of contingency table analysis. South Korean citizens' evaluation of their own country's response to the pandemic varied according to generations, $\chi^2 = 16.280$, $p = 0.003$. The percentage of favorable evaluations of South Korea's anti-pandemic response was higher among the older generations than among their younger counterparts. Among respondents over age 50, 55.11% viewed South Korea's anti-pandemic response as successful, while 23.92% considered it unsuccessful. In contrast, among respondents between 18 and 30 years old, 37.84% evaluated South Korea's response as successful, and 35.14% as unsuccessful, which was more even.

Although South Korean citizens evaluated China's anti-pandemic response unfavorably for the most part, an intergenerational difference was apparent in the evaluations, $\chi^2 = 50.662$, $p < 0.001$. The older generations evaluated China's response more favorably than the younger ones. Among respondents who were over 50 years old, 50.27% viewed China's response as unsuccessful. This

Table 9.3 Variations of South Korean citizens' evaluations of domestic and foreign responses to the pandemic across different generations

		Evaluations of the responses to the pandemic									*Total*
		China			*Japan*			*South Korea*			
		Unsuccessful	*Neutral*	*Successful*	*Unsuccessful*	*Neutral*	*Successful*	*Unsuccessful*	*Neutral*	*Successful*	
Generations	18–30	115 (77.70%)	21 (14.19%)	12 (8.11%)	83 (56.08%)	39 (26.35%)	26 (17.57%)	52 (35.14%)	40 (27.03%)	56 (37.84%)	148 (17.05%)
	31–50	243 (69.83%)	71 (20.40%)	34 (9.77%)	244 (70.11%)	77 (22.13%)	27 (7.76%)	98 (28.16%)	95 (27.30%)	155 (44.54%)	348 (40.09%)
	51–	187 (50.27%)	103 (27.69%)	82 (22.04%)	214 (57.53%)	91 (24.46%)	67 (18.01%)	89 (23.92%)	78 (20.97%)	205 (55.11%)	372 (42.86%)
	Total	545 (62.79%)	195 (22.47%)	128 (14.75%)	541 (62.33%)	207 (23.85%)	120 (13.82%)	239 (27.53%)	213 (24.54%)	416 (47.93%)	868 (100%)

percentage rose to 77.70% among respondents from 18 to 30 years old. Younger South Koreans expressed greater disapproval of China's anti-pandemic response.

South Korean citizens' evaluations of Japan's anti-pandemic response also varied across generations, $\chi^2 = 20.046$, $p < 0.001$. Specifically, 56.08% of respondents between 18 and 30 years old and 57.53% of respondents over age 50 evaluated Japan's anti-pandemic response unfavorably, whereas 70.11% of respondents between 31 and 50 years old viewed Japan's response as unsuccessful. Middle-aged South Koreans evaluated Japan's response more negatively than did other age groups.

Some conclusions can be drawn from the aforementioned results. South Korean citizens' evaluations of their domestic and neighboring countries' responses to the pandemic varied significantly across generations. The under-30 generation expressed greater disapproval of China's response, and the 31–50 generation expressed greater disapproval of Japan's response. Finally, the over-51 generation expressed greater approval of their own country's response to the pandemic. Although younger South Koreans negatively evaluated China's and Japan's anti-COVID responses, they viewed China much less favorably.

Multivariate regression analysis was performed to examine the relationship between South Korean citizens' access to information and their evaluations of domestic and neighboring countries' responses to the pandemic. Figure 9.3 presents the major results regarding the effects of access to information, omitting the display of the demographic variables.

Access to information from television was positively associated with favorable evaluations of South Korea's response ($b = 0.117$, $p = 0.006$), with which information from newspapers was negatively associated ($b = -0.152$, $p < 0.001$). Information from interpersonal networks did not significantly affect evaluations of South Korea's domestic response to the pandemic. In terms of evaluation of China's response, access to information from newspapers and television was positively associated with approval of China's response ($b = 0.085$, $p = 0.022$; $b = 0.083$, $p = 0.046$), with which internet use was negatively associated ($b = -0.158$, $p < 0.001$). In terms of evaluations of Japan's anti-pandemic response, access to information from newspapers and social media was positively associated with approval of Japan's response ($b = 0.099$, $p = 0.009$; $b = 0.179$, $p < 0.001$), with which internet use was negatively associated ($b = -0.178$, $p < 0.001$). In addition, information from colleagues was negatively associated with South Korean citizens' approval of Japan's response to the pandemic ($b = -0.121$, $p = 0.008$).

The findings from South Korea have several implications. First, access to pandemic-related information from newspapers was positively associated with approval of China's and Japan's anti-pandemic response but negatively associated with approval of their domestic response. The results did not negate South Korean newspapers' unfavorable coverage of China and Japan. As newspapers were the least frequently used approach to acquiring information on the pandemic in South Korea (see Figure 9.1), their positive influence on approval of China and Japan would be limited. Conservative newspapers' negative views on China reflected their discontent with the Moon administration. For example, the newspaper *Chosun* criticized the Moon administration for turning a blind eye to China's cover-up of the outbreak and ignoring the suffering of the South Korean people (Chung et al., 2021). This might explain the reasons for South Korean citizens' negative association of access to information by newspapers and disapproval of the domestic response to the pandemic. Second, internet use was significantly related to disapproval of China's and Japan's anti-pandemic measures. Figure 9.1 reveals that the internet was the information source on the COVID-19 pandemic most frequently used by South Koreans. Online information in South Korea might be more negative about the two countries. This could explain the unfavorable evaluations of China and Japan.

Conclusion

This chapter analyzed Chinese, Japanese, and South Korean citizens' evaluations of their domestic and neighboring countries' anti-pandemic responses through examining their sources of information. Citizens in these three East Asian countries had distinct patterns of evaluations of each country's response. Japanese people were most critical and disapproving of all three countries' responses. They did not even favorably evaluate Japan. Researchers have assumed that citizens in post-materialist societies are critical of the authorities (Dalton and Welzel, 2014; Inglehart and Welzel, 2005; Norris, 1999). Japan was the only country among the three surveyed East Asian countries that showed such a critical tendency. Chinese and South Korean citizens showed favoritism to their own countries. They perceived the domestic response to the pandemic as successful but evaluated neighboring countries unfavorably. Although ingroup favoritism was found in the case of both China and South Korea, Chinese citizens showed extraordinarily high levels of approval of China. Specifically, 94.70% of Chinese respondents viewed their country's response to the pandemic as successful during the first two years after the initial outbreak of COVID-19. This assessment of the Chinese people contrasts with the Pew Research Center's finding that China's pandemic response was widely regarded as unfavorable outside of China (Silver et al., 2020). This mentality is prevalent among Chinese citizens. In fact, studies show extraordinarily high domestic levels of approval of China in other fields such as trust in government, the country's level of democratic development, and the favorable influence of the country's rise on the world (Shi, 2008; Sonoda, 2014; Wu and Wilkes, 2018; Zhai, 2018, 2023a). Chinese people's national pride, the state's propaganda, and the state-censored information environment may account for this phenomenon.

The present study examined the information environment of the three countries, through which people accessed information on the COVID-19 pandemic. The information environment comprises the media and interpersonal networks. Our survey shows that television, the internet, and family were the primary sources of information for people in the three countries. On the one hand, people depend on the internet to access information in the digital era. On the other hand, different types of mass media play distinct roles in information provision during the pandemic. The present study found that, although the influence of newspapers declined, television maintained its influence. Moreover, Chinese, Japanese, and South Koreans also used interpersonal networks to acquire information. Frequency of access to information from family, friends, and colleagues reflects the characteristics of personal relationships in the three countries. Japanese people rarely obtained information on the pandemic from colleagues. However, South Korean people accessed information from colleagues less frequently than from family members and friends. In contrast, behavioral modes between different personal relationships in China are less differentiated than those in Japan and South Korea. As a result, the frequency with which Chinese people accessed information about the COVID-19 pandemic from colleagues was similar to the frequency with which they accessed information from family members and friends. These results indicate that despite the three countries having a common cultural tradition, the difference in social relationships between them is also significant.

The empirical analysis demonstrated that access to information affected people's evaluations of their domestic and neighboring countries' anti-pandemic responses in China, Japan, and South Korea. The effect of information varied according to different information sources and the specific country.

In China, access to information from television and the internet was positively associated with favorable evaluations of China's anti-pandemic response. The positive effect of television was less surprising, as television agencies in China are run by the government at different levels. Mass media is not independent from the state and is no more than a means of propaganda. The internet is often considered to provide more diverse information than traditional media, and various criticisms of the authorities are indeed made online (Tang and Huhe, 2020; Xiang and Hmielowski, 2017; Yang, 2013). In terms of food safety, corruption, and environmental pollution, internet use was often negatively associated with evaluations of the authorities. The positive effect of access to information from the internet on Chinese citizens' evaluations of the country indicates the state's increasing control of the internet. The Chinese authorities spare little effort when it comes to internet surveillance and censorship (Chang and Lin, 2020; Goldsmith and Wu, 2006; Xiao, 2019). The Great Firewall blocks domestic access to Google, Facebook, Instagram, Twitter, and many Western news platforms. The Chinese state has adapted to employ the new digital media for propaganda purposes and prevent it from becoming a platform for opposition forces. For example, pro-government videos and comments flooded the Chinese internet, and negative comments about China or the Chinese Communist Party were quickly detected and deleted by surveillance machines. The state seeks to employ the internet as an instrument to intensify its control over people and ensure regime stability. The favorable effect of access to online information on approval of the country's anti-pandemic response signals this change in China's internet environment.

A phenomenon worth noting in Japan and South Korea was the negative effect of the internet on evaluations of neighboring countries' responses to the pandemic. In Japan, access to information on the internet was related to disapproval of South Korea's response to the pandemic. In South Korea, internet use was related to disapproval of China's and Japan's responses. The internet connects people from different countries, creating expectations that it will facilitate the formation of a global village. However, the internet became replete with racism and xenophobic narratives, and it became a platform for the expression of nationalist sentiments. Political unrest in East Asia often arouses conflict in real life, and the debate continues in the virtual world. Nationalist netizens in the three countries exchange vitriol and insults on the internet (Sasada, 2006; Takahara, 2006). Curran et al. (2013) found that online news was strongly nation-centered. Other studies found that internet use intensified national identification by facilitating the formation and dissemination of nationalist discourse (Eriksen, 2007; Miller and Slater, 2000). Nationalist sentiment is usually related to disapproval of other nations. The findings regarding the negative relationships between access to information on the internet and unfavorable evaluations of neighboring countries' anti-pandemic responses revealed the existence of more negative online information about foreign countries than did other information sources. This characteristic indicates that the internet plays a complex role in globalization.

Although interpersonal networks are important means of access to information, this information source rarely affected people's evaluations of their domestic and neighboring countries' anti-pandemic responses in the three countries. The only significant effect was observed in the relationship between South Korean citizens' access to information from colleagues and their evaluations of Japan's response. South Korea has a working atmosphere that is distinct from those of China and Japan. Japanese people rarely accessed information on the pandemic from colleagues, while Chinese people exchanged and shared information on the pandemic with colleagues at a level similar to family members and friends. South Korean people were less likely to access information on the pandemic from colleagues than through other personal networks such as friends. Negative information on Japan's response to the pandemic might have been circulating in South Korea's workplaces. Therefore, access to information from colleagues was negatively associated with disapproval of Japan's anti-pandemic response.

In summary, this chapter identified the characteristics of access to information on COVID-19 in China, Japan, and South Korea, as well as the relationship between access to information and approval of domestic and neighboring countries' anti-pandemic responses. Information is an important cause of (dis)approval of a country's anti-pandemic response. Comparison with the performance of other countries in infection prevention and control can affect people's attitudes toward the domestic situation (Jo and Chang, 2020). States may intentionally manipulate information about other countries to shape public evaluations of their own anti-pandemic performance. Future research should further examine factors that may mediate information sources and evaluations of the country's response. For example, the credibility of information sources, the political slants of the media agencies, and the degree of people's vigilance toward fake news and misinformation may affect the relationship between access to information and the approval of domestic and foreign countries' responses. In addition, future research should consider some pre-existing values or attitudes toward the domestic governments and foreign countries.

References

Anderson, Benedict. 2006. *Imagined Communities: Reflections on the Origin and Spread of Nationalism*. London, England: Verso.

Bednarek, Monika and Helen Caple. 2017. *The Discourse of News Values: How News Organizations Create Newsworthiness*. Oxford: Oxford University Press.

Boase, Jeffrey and Ken'ichi Ikeda. 2012. Core discussion networks in Japan and America. *Human Communication Research* 38(1): 95–119.

Castles, Stephen. 2011. Globalization, ethnic identity and the integration crisis. *Ethnicities* 11(1): 23–26.

Chang, Chun-Chih and Thung-Hong Lin. 2020. Autocracy login: Internet censorship and civil society in the digital age. *Democratization* 27(5): 874–895.

Chi, Eunju. 2012. The Chinese government's responses to use of the Internet. *Asian Perspective* 36(3): 387–409.

Chrisman, Robert. 2008. Globalization and the media industry. *The Black Scholar* 43(3): 74–77.

Chung, Angie Y., Hyerim Jo, Ji-won Lee, and Fan Yang. 2021. COVID-19 and the political framing of China, nationalism, and borders in the U.S. and South Korean news media. *Sociological Perspectives* 64(5): 747–764.

Chung, Regina Wai-man and King-wa Fu. 2022. Tweets and memories: Chinese censors come after me. Forbidden voices of the 1989 Tiananmen Square massacre on Sina Weibo, 2012–2018. *Journal of Contemporary China* 31(134): 319–334.

Curran, James, Sharon Coen, Toril Aalberg, Kaori Hayashi, Paul K. Jones, Sergio Splendore, Stylianos Papathanassopoulos, David Rowe, and Rod Tiffen. 2013. Internet revolution revisited: A comparative study of online news. *Media, Culture and Society* 35(7): 880–897.

Dalton, Russell J. and Christian Welzel. 2014. *The Civic Culture Transformed: From Allegiant to Assertive Citizens*. Cambridge: Cambridge University Press.

Efferson, Charles, Rafael Lalive, and Ernst Fehr. 2008. The coevolution of cultural groups and ingroup favoritism. *Science* 321(5897): 1844–1849.

Eriksen, Thomas. 2007. Nationalism and the internet. *Nations and Nationalism* 13(1): 1–17.

First, Jennifer M., Haejung Shin, Yerina S. Ranjit, and J. Brian Houston. 2021. COVID-19 stress and depression: Examining social media, traditional media, and interpersonal communication. *Journal of Loss and Trauma* 26(2): 101–115.

Fisher, Ronald. 1990. *The Social Psychology of Intergroup and International Conflict Resolution*. New York: Springer-Verlag.

Fiss, Peer C. and Paul M. Hirsch. 2005. The discourse of globalization: Framing and sensemaking of an emerging concept. *American Sociological Review* 70(1): 29–52.

Fukasawa, Maiko, Norito Kawakami, Chihiro Nakayama, and Seiji Yasumura. 2021. Relationship between use of media and radiation anxiety among the residents of Fukushima 5.5 years after the nuclear power plant accident. *Disaster Medicine and Public Health Preparedness* 15(1): 42–49.

Gao, Junling, Pinpin Zheng, Yingnan Jia, Hao Chen, Yimeng Mao, Suhong Chen, Yi Wang, Hua Fu, and Junming Dai. 2020. Mental health problems and social media exposure during COVID-19 outbreak. *PLoS One* 15(4): e0231924.

Goldsmith, Jack and Tim Wu. 2006. *Who Controls the Internet? Illusions of a Borderless World*. Oxford: Oxford University Press.

Guo, Steve and Dan Wang. 2021. News production and construal level: A comparative analysis of the press coverage of China's Belt and Road Initiative. *Chinese Journal of Communication* 14(2): 211–230.

Han, Guanghua and Yida Zhai. 2022. Perceptions of food safety, access to information, and political trust in China. *Chinese Journal of Communication* 15(4): 534–557.

Ikeda, Ken'ichi and Jeffrey Boase. 2011. Multiple discussion networks and their consequence for political participation. *Communication Research* 38(5): 660–683.

Ikeda, Ken'ichi and Sean E. Richey. 2005. Japanese network capital: The impact of social networks on Japanese political participation. *Political Behavior* 27: 239–260.

Inglehart, Ronald and Christian Welzel. 2005. *Modernization, Cultural Change, and Democracy: The Human Development Sequence*. Cambridge: Cambridge University Press.

Jang, Kyungeun and Young Min Baek. 2019. When information from public health officials is untrustworthy: The use of online news, interpersonal networks, and social media during the MERS outbreak in South Korea. *Health Communication* 34(9): 991–998.

Jo, Wonkwang and Dukjin Chang. 2020. Political consequences of COVID-19 and media framing in South Korea. *Frontiers in Public Health* 8: 425.

Lee, Hocheol, Eun Bi Noh, Sea Hwan Choi, Bo Zhao, and Eun Woo Nam. 2020. Determining public opinion of the COVID-19 pandemic in South Korea and Japan: Social network mining on Twitter. *Healthcare Informatics Research* 26(4): 335–343.

Miller, Daniel and Don Slater. 2000. *The Internet: An Ethnographic Approach*. Oxford: Berg.

Monge, Peter R and Noshir Contractor. 2003. *Theories of Communication Networks*. Oxford: Oxford University Press.

Morris, Jonathan S. 2007. Slanted objectivity? Perceived media bias, cable news exposure, and political attitudes. *Social Science Quarterly* 88(3): 707–728.

Norris, Pippa. 1999. *Critical Citizens: Support for Democratic Government*. Oxford: Oxford University Press.

Parvin, Gulsan Ara, Md. Habibur Rahman, S.M. Reazul Ahsan, Md. Anwarul Abedin, and Mrittika Basu. 2022. Media discourse in China and Japan on the COVID-19 pandemic: Comparative analysis of the first three months. *Journal of Information, Communication and Ethics in Society* 20(2): 308–328.

Pye, Lucian W. 1968. *The Spirit of Chinese Politics*. Cambridge, MA: The MIT Press.

Richey, Sean and Ken'ichi Ikeda. 2006. The influence of political discussion on policy preference: A comparison of the United States and Japan. *Japanese Journal of Political Science* 7(3): 273–288.

Romano, Angelo, Daniel Balliet, Toshio Yamagishi, and James H. Liu. 2017. Parochial trust and cooperation across 17 societies. *Proceedings of the National Academy of Sciences* 114(48): 12702–12707.

Sasada, Hironori. 2006. Youth and nationalism in Japan. *SAIS Review* 26: 109–122.

Scheufele, Dietram A., Matthew C. Nisbet, Dominique Brossard, and Erik C. Nisbet. 2004. Social structure and citizenship: Examining the impacts of social setting, network heterogeneity, and information variables on political participation. *Political Communication* 21(3): 315–338.

Shi, Tianjian. 2008. China: Democratic values supporting an authoritarian system. In Yunhan Chu, Larry Diamond, Andrew J. Nathan, and Doh Chull Shin (eds.), *How East Asians View Democracy*. New York: Columbia University Press, pp. 209–237.

Silver, Laura, Kat Devlin, and Christine Huang. 2020. Unfavorable views of China reach historic highs in many countries. Pew Research Center, October 6, 2020. www.pewresearch.org/global/2020/10/06/unfavorable-views-of-china-reach-historic-highs-in-many-countries/

Silver, Roxane Cohen, E Alison Holman, Judith Pizarro Andersen, Michael Poulin, Daniel N. McIntosh, and Virginia Gil-Rivas. 2013. Mental- and physical-health effects of acute exposure to media images of the September 11, 2001, attacks and the Iraq War. *Psychological Science* 24(9): 1623–1634.

Sonoda, Shigeto. 2014. What does China's rise bring about? *Ajia Jiho [Asian Times]* 45: 36–57 (in Japanese).

Spence, Patric R., Ken Lachlan, Jennifer M. Burke, and Matthew W. Seeger. 2007. Media use and information needs of the disabled during a natural disaster. *Journal of Health Care for the Poor and Underserved* 18(2): 394–404.

Tai, Qiuqing. 2014. China's media censorship: A dynamic and diversified regime. *Journal of East Asian Studies* 14(2): 185–210.

Tajfel, Henri. 1974. Social identity and intergroup behavior. *Social Science Information* 13(2): 65–93.

Tajfel, Henri. 1982. Social psychology of intergroup relations. *Annual Review of Psychology* 33: 1–39.

Tajfel, Henri and John Turner. 1986. An integrative theory of intergroup conflict. In Stephen Worchel and William G. Austin (eds.), *Psychology of Intergroup Relations*. Chicago, IL: Nelson-Hall, pp. 2–24.

Takahara, Motoaki. 2006. *The Era of Unstable Nationalism: Why the Japanese, Korean, and Chinese Internet Generation Detest Each Other*. Tokyo: Yosensha (in Japanese).

Tang, Min and Narisong Huhe. 2020. Parsing the effect of the internet on regime support in China. *Government and Opposition* 55(1): 130–146.

The Genron NPO. 2021. Opinion polls. www.genron-npo.net/en/opinion_polls/

Thompson, Rebecca R., Dana Rose Garfin, E. Alison Holman, and Roxane Cohen Silver. 2017. Distress, worry, and functioning following a global health crisis: A national study of Americans' responses to Ebola. *Clinical Psychological Science* 5(3): 513–521.

Weimann, Gabriel. 1983. The strength of weak conversational ties in the flow of information and influence. *Social Networks* 5(3): 245–267.

Wu, Cary and Rima Wilkes. 2018. Local-national political trust patterns: Why China is an exception. *International Political Science Review* 39(4): 436–454.

Xiang, Jun and Jay D. Hmielowski. 2017. Alternative views and eroding support: The conditional Indirect effects of foreign media and Internet use on regime support in China. *International Journal of Public Opinion Research* 29(3): 406–425.

Xiao, Qiang. 2019. The road to digital unfreedom: President Xi's surveillance state. *Journal of Democracy* 30(1): 53–67.

Yang, Guobin. 2013. Contesting food safety in the Chinese media: Between hegemony and counter-hegemony. *The China Quarterly* 214: 337–355.

Yang, Yuan, Min Tang, Wang Zhou, and Narisong Huhe. 2014. The effect of media use on institutional trust in China. *Problems of Post-Communism* 61(3): 45–56.

Zhai, Yida. 2018. The gap in viewing China's rise between Chinese youth and their Asian counterparts. *Journal of Contemporary China* 27(114): 848–866.

Zhai, Yida. 2021. The role of online social capital in the relationship between Internet use and self-worth. *Current Psychology* 40(5): 2073–2082.

Zhai, Yida. 2023a. Public opinion in a rising power: National and international orientations among the Chinese public. *Journal of East Asian Studies* 23(1): 71–94.

Zhai, Yida. 2023b. The politics of COVID-19: The political logic of China's Zero-COVID policy. *Journal of Contemporary Asia* 53(5): 869–886.

Zhai, Yida. 2024. The COVID-19 pandemic and popular confidence in democracy: Evidence from China, Japan, and South Korea. *Democratization*, DOI: 10.1080/13510347.2024.2355245.

Zhai, Yida, Li Ying Chong, Yunzhe Liu, Shuting Yang, and Changfa Song. 2022. Social dominance orientation, right-wing authoritarianism, and political attitudes toward governmental performance during the COVID-19 pandemic. *Analyses of Social Issues and Public Policy* 22(1): 150–167.

Zhao, Bo, Mahyeon Kim, and Eun Woo Nam. 2021. Information disclosure contents of the COVID-19 data dashboard websites for South Korea, China, and Japan: A comparative study. *Healthcare* 9(11): 1487.

Zhu, Ying. 2014. *Two Billion Eyes: The Story of China Central Television*. New York: The New Press.

Index

Note 1: Entries in bold refer to tables, entries in italics refer to figures.
Note 2: "Korea" refers to South Korea

For Product Safety Concerns and Information please contact our EU representative GPSR@taylorandfrancis.com
Taylor & Francis Verlag GmbH, Kaufingerstraße 24, 80331 München, Germany

www.ingramcontent.com/pod-product-compliance
Lightning Source LLC
LaVergne TN
LVHW010902110826
845149LV00005B/1447

* 9 7 8 1 0 3 2 8 0 0 6 2 2 *